Understanding &
Working with
Substance Misusers

'Building on the principles of motivational interviewing and a whole systems approach, Aaron Pycroft masterfully addresses the complexity of substance misuse. Educators in the helping professions and addiction experts will find Understanding and Working with Substance Misusers *a highly informative and thought-provoking resource.*'
Katherine van Wormer, co-author of *Addiction Treatment: A Strengths Perspective*, Professor of Social Work, University of Northern Iowa

'In addressing the essentials of understanding substance use and misuse, Aaron Pycroft has provided a comprehensive approach whilst remaining grounded in evidence.'
Dr Peter Phillips, City University London

Understanding & Working with Substance Misusers

Aaron Pycroft

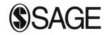

Los Angeles | London | New Delhi
Singapore | Washington DC

First published 2010

SAGE Publications Ltd
1 Oliver's Yard
55 City Road
London EC1Y 1SP

SAGE Publications Inc.
2455 Teller Road
Thousand Oaks, California 91320

SAGE Publications India Pvt Ltd
B 1/I 1 Mohan Cooperative Industrial Area
Mathura Road
New Delhi 110 044

SAGE Publications Asia-Pacific Pte Ltd
33 Pekin Street #02-01
Far East Square
Singapore 048763

Library of Congress Control Number: 2009940797

British Library Cataloguing in Publication data

A catalogue record for this book is available from the British Library

ISBN 978-1-84787-261-6
ISBN 978-1-84787-262-3 (pbk)

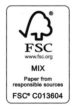

Typeset by C&M Digitals (P) Ltd, Chennai, India
Printed by CPI Antony Rowe, Chippenham, Wiltshire
Printed on paper from sustainable resources

As ever my work is dedicated to my beautiful and wonderful family
Nicky, Samuel, Barnabas and Lydia

Contents

List of Tables and Figures

Author Information

Aaron Pycroft is a Senior Lecturer in Addition Studies in the Institute of Criminal Justice Studies at the University of Portsmouth, where he has developed both undergraduate and postgraduate courses in the study of substance misuse. Prior to this Aaron worked for 15 years as a practitioner and senior manager in providing detox, rehab and other support services for substance misusers. He is actively engaged in researching, writing, knowledge transfer and training activities in this area of work. Aaron's primary interest is in the application of complexity theory to the study of addiction and treatment interventions and his book co-edited with Dennis Gough, *Multi-Agency Working: Control and Care in Contemporary Correctional Practice* (2010), is published by Policy Press.

Preface and Acknowledgements

In academia there would appear to be two types of book: one type written by academics for academics, and the other by academics and/or practitioners for students taking degree courses and vocational qualifications. Very often one set of books does not inform the other, and as a consequence of this much of the knowledge that is being developed and discussed in the academy does not make its way into professional practice. In the academy itself the separation of disciplines and everything from the 'unitisation' of curricula through to the way that research is funded leaves people working in their own intellectual silos and perhaps rarely influenced by voices from the 'real world' who are experiencing and dealing with the issues under discussion.

This book is an attempt to address some of those issues, and it arises out of a number of key influences all of which are very strikingly similar albeit in different contexts: firstly my practice experience in trying to work with people who have substance misuse problems; secondly in trying to persuade commissioners and decision makers to engage in more sophisticated and joined up thinking about the delivery of services; and thirdly, since taking up an academic post, in trying to find a way of teaching these issues which are cross cutting and also require the academy to engage in more joined up thinking.

Recently a colleague, on asking me how the book was coming along, remarked that he thought that this was a particularly difficult one to write given that the scope is to try and make sense of the biopsychosocial paradigm of addiction. The colleague thought that there was an inherent risk in trying to cover too much; by attempting to cover the key themes from biology, psychology and social context how can one book do justice to such huge areas of scientific endeavour; it may be that subject specific practitioners or academics are left disappointed by a perceived lack of depth? Whilst acknowledging that danger my purpose is: firstly to try and make biopsychosociality comprehensible to students, practitioners and fellow academics; and secondly to argue that complexity theory provides us with a cross-disciplinary framework to understand and work with these issues. It is my contention that the study of complexity allows us to peer inside and start to comprehend the 'black box' of treatment and its equivocal outcomes. In making these arguments I am trying to develop some relatively new and emergent ideas in an accessible way.

This book represents a long journey in the study of addiction which has lasted over 20 years. I came into it by 'accident' but it is a journey that still keeps me fascinated and enthralled, almost addicted! Between 1989 and 2003 I had the privilege of working with some remarkable people at the Society of St Dismas which latterly became the Two Saints Housing Association. In 1989 this organisation established the first purpose built community alcohol detox and aftercare centre in the country which is now sadly closed (an apt lesson in the impact of policy decisions and the intended and unintended consequences that go with them). In working with the staff and service users I learnt about addiction and was given the opportunity to grow and develop as a practitioner, manager, academic and trainer. In that respect this book owes a great deal not only to all of my colleagues during that time, but also to the service users. I have always been impressed and humbled by the sheer tenacity of people with severe problems, who against the odds strive for a better future. If there is one thing that I have learnt it is to listen to what a service user is saying about their situation – they are the expert, they have a great deal of knowledge and often what they need is help with human and material resources to implement change.

In writing this book I have to thank my colleagues at the Institute of Criminal Justice Studies at the University of Portsmouth for their support and encouragement. I would like to thank Mike Nash and Mark Mitchell for alleviating me of marking and other such responsibilities at some important stages of writing. Also thanks goes to Suzie Clift for reviewing chapters and making helpful suggestions and comments as I have gone along, and also for finding the book useful enough to endorse. Outside of ICJS I need to acknowledge and thank my old and dear friend Paul Jennings for getting me to think about the implications of evolutionary theory for human behaviour and for helping me out with some of the maths involved in complexity theory. Despite all of this generous help and support any errors empirical or conceptual are of course entirely my own. A really big 'thank you' also goes to Fiona for agreeing to be interviewed for the final chapter and for sharing an incredible journey to recovery. Finally I need to thank Zoe Elliot-Fawcett, Alison Poyner and Emma Paterson at Sage for their support and patience throughout this project.

List of Abbreviations

AA – Alcoholics Anonymous
ACMD – Advisory Council for the Misuse of Drugs
ADS – Alcohol Dependence Syndrome
AIDS – Acquired Immuno Deficiency Syndrome
ANARP – Alcohol Needs Assessment Research Project
ATR – Alcohol Treatment Requirement
AUD – Alcohol Use Disorder
AVE – Abstinence Violation Effect
CA – Cellular Automata
CADT – Community Alcohol and Drug Team
CBT – Cognitive Behavioural Therapy
CMDA – Cortico-mesolimbic dopamine system
DAT – Drug Action Team
DNA – Deoxyribonucleic Acid
DOH – Department of Health
DRR – Drug Rehabilitation Requirement
DSM-IV – *Diagnostic and Statistical Manual* (4th edition)
DTORS – Drug Treatment Outcome Research Study
EMCDDA – European Monitoring Centre for Drugs and Drug Addiction
ESPAD – European Schools Project on Alcohol and Drugs
HAV – Hepatitis A Virus
HBV – Hepatitis B Virus
HCV – Hepatitis C Virus
HIV – Human Immune Deficiency Virus
ICD -10 – *International Classification of Diseases* (10th edition)
IDU – Injecting Drug User
IOM – Institute of Medicine
LAAM – Levo-alpha-acetyl-methadol
MET – Motivational Enhancement Therapy
MI – Motivational Interviewing

MOC – Models of Care
MoCAM – Models of Care for Alcohol Misusers
NA – Narcotics Anonymous
NTA – National Treatment Agency for Substance Misuse
NTORS – National Treatment Outcome Research Study
RIOTT – Randomised Injectable Opioid Treatment Trial
RCT – Randomised Controlled Trial
SBNT – Social Behaviour and Network Therapy
TSF – Twelve Step Facilitation
TTM – Trans Theoretical Model of Change
UKATT – United Kingdom Alcohol Treatment Trial
UN – United Nations
UNODC – United Nations Office of Drugs and Crime
WHO – World Health Organisation

Introduction

This book is about human beings: people, me and you. It is about firstly what happens when we use certain substances called 'drugs' that are described as 'psychoactive', and secondly about some of the consequences that can occur biologically, psychologically and socially as a result of that drug use. The use of psychoactive substances, whether extracted from nature in their raw state or treated to increase their potency, has been prevalent in most cultures since the dawn of time. The use of these substances, and the pleasures and pains that are experienced therein, present some real challenges for individuals and society in general. All of us experience to differing degrees, compulsions, addictions and habitual behaviours, some of which may be as a result of evolutionary processes. The interdisciplinary nature of these problems can also create real challenges for students and professionals who study and work in this area.

Different cultures have a differing spectrum of drug use which sees different people using different drugs to differing degrees; some of whom will not experience any difficulties related to that usage, some of whom will move in and out of problem areas, and some of whom will experience apparently chronic and intractable problems. This book is primarily concerned with the idea of 'addiction' and the bringing together of ideas from the three areas of biology, psychology and the study of social context, and to make accessible some of the key issues involved in what is called the 'biopsychosocial paradigm'. It is also about relating ideas of addiction to a policy, public health, and treatment and prevention agenda. As the use of drugs both licit and illicit has become a major issue particularly for industrialised countries, and our understanding of the issues has become more dimensional in nature, then more and more professional groups are required to have an understanding of drug use and its related issues. This book aims to bring together some of the issues from different academic and practitioner backgrounds to inform this important work.

Over recent years the developing consensus around biopsychosociality which hypothesises that addiction is about more than the sum of its individual parts (Lindstrom, 1992; Lende and Smith, 2002) has challenged academics and practitioners to break out of their traditional areas of study, and to start to become acquainted with these other disciplines. One of the key messages of this book is that an acceptance of complexity cannot be avoided; in fact it will be argued that it is precisely by addressing the issues of complexity that arise from complex interactions that we can make further progress in our ethical awareness, and theory building in the development of more effective interventions, for the alleviation of suffering.

In the industrialised world the expansion of psychotherapy, self-help books and groups, dieting programmes, drug and alcohol programmes, and gyms shows that undesirable behaviour is a part of the human condition and that many of us are trying (usually unsuccessfully) to change our thoughts, feelings and actions. A key aim of this book is to place behaviour around psychoactive substances within the range of behaviours that we should expect from human beings. At the time of writing the world is celebrating the bicentenary of Charles Darwin, and his legacy of the role of evolution in shaping the world and our place in it is as applicable to drug use as it is to all other aspects of human behaviour.

Once we start to consider questions within an evolutionary context and look at issues in new ways using developments in modern science and philosophy then we might agree with Orford (1990: 211) that given the existence of the biopsychosocial paradigm this may 'be of particular significance in the study of human kind'. This mystery and intrigue can provide us with the motivation to pursue solutions which are particularly important when acknowledging some of the serious problems involved in an approach that is necessarily multi-disciplinary (by my estimation economics, history, politics, social policy and public health, biology and technology have already been referenced at the very least) for both academics and practitioners. It is essential, whether you are theory building, researching, or practically helping people, to break out of the comfort blanket of your subject or professional specialism (see Chick, 2002: 474) and to collaborate across the broad areas of biology, psychology and sociology. In this respect because 'there's no one lead discipline that is committed to the drug abuse problem comprehensively' (Edwards, 2002: 37), then there are important challenges for practitioners who decide upon and deliver interventions and also for commissioners and politicians who plan and fund services.

Key questions

This book is very much focused upon the idea of 'addiction', addiction to drugs and what this means and in what senses our understanding of it might be useful in helping people who are suffering from it. However, as we shall see, addiction very much arises from the interactions of the supply and availability of drugs, the drugs themselves, the make up of the individual, and the context in which the drugs are used. It is important to acknowledge that there is a process leading to addiction and that in terms of prevention, alleviation and treatment that a range of interventions may be required at different levels.

This book will therefore outline the context for the supply and prevalence of substance use as necessary background for understanding some of the primary reasons why addiction to substances arises. Whilst there are a plethora of questions to be asked concerning the nature of drug use, the questions that are most frequently raised in the field of addiction are as follows:

1 Why do people begin using drugs?
2 How and why does drug use escalate to misuse?
3 Why does this continue despite severe consequences?
4 Why and how do people stop or modify their drug taking?
5 Why is addiction so difficult to treat?
6 Why is it the norm for people to relapse after a period of abstinence or controlled use?
7 What is the relationship between addiction and multiple problem areas?
8 Why is there such a common occurrence with psychiatric disorders?
   (Adapted from Lindstrom, 1992/Bickell and Potenza, 2006)

Questions such as these of course then beg a whole series of questions of their own in the demand for conceptual clarity and theoretical consistency, as well as practical utility. In the course of the book there will be an attempt to address all of these questions at an introductory level and in a way that is accessible to a range of readers from diverse academic and practitioner backgrounds.

Key issues

In seeking an understanding of these important and ubiquitous issues then experience shows us that we have to, in the first instance, accept that complexity is the *sine qua non* in this field and that, within that complexity, there are a number of key realities that should be acknowledged:

1 Virtually every human being at some stage during their life will use a psychoactive substance, legal or illegal. Currently the mostly widely used substances are caffeine, alcohol and nicotine.
2 Attitudes, and societal and policy responses, have changed over the course of time as to which drugs should be freely available, controlled or banned. Consequently the

language and labels used to describe, analyse and ascribe the morality of actions change as well.

3   There is a nexus of issues and problems that can become involved with the use of substances, even legal ones, that may either be bio-psychological in nature (for example, severe withdrawal symptoms from alcohol or heroin) or socially constructed (for example, making the use of certain drugs a criminal offence in its own right). It is important not to confuse the two sets of issues. Therefore our starting point should not be legality, or the contemporaneous status quo, but the evidence available for the nature of particular drugs and the nature of their benefits and harms. This has to involve a hard-nosed and realistic comparison of the nature of risk for each substance.

4   There are no simple solutions to complex problems, and as we look in more detail at the nature of complexity itself we will see that the solutions that may seem grounded in common sense (and are often proclaimed by politicians and the media) such as 'more treatment is needed' or 'just say no to drugs' or 'we need to legalise drugs' are not necessarily evidence based, and may even be counterproductive. There are always intended and unintended outcomes from decisions at any level, whether clinical or policy led.

5   Scientific research, academic debate, and the formulation of policies are important in finding solutions to some of society's most intractable problems. But the focus of these endeavours are human beings who whether through their drug use, or because they are living with or caring for someone who uses drugs, or because they live in the same community as a drug user may well be suffering physical, psychological and social disadvantage. Any attempt to alleviate this suffering ultimately has to be person and community centred, and should listen to the voices of the people who are suffering. An individual's experience of drug use and the effect of drug use will have commonalities as well as differences with other people's drug use, and each needs to be listened to in informing policy and practice.

Language and labels

Semantics have played an important and controversial role in the study of the use of psychoactive substances. A part of the difficulty in this area comes from the differentiations made between which drugs are legal or illegal, or between drugs and associated behaviours which are seen to be worthy of moral condemnation. This can lead to confusion and disagreement even amongst the experts; for example, Goldstein (2001: 4) states 'incorrect use of language shapes incorrect ways of thinking', whereas Edwards and Gross (1976) argue that whether drug dependence should be seen as a syndrome or a disease is largely semantic. However, language is important in defining problems, attributing notions of responsibility, and planning interventions. Within sociology labelling theory (see Newburn, 2007) has made an important contribution to our understanding of how people and communities are excluded and included from wider society and its benefits through the imposition of labels.

For Babor (1992) any system of definition or classification should be convenient to work with, allow inferences to be made about underlying causes, provide for theory building and research, and facilitate communication between academics, researchers and practitioners. Following on from Babor's approach and unless otherwise stated this book will use the terms 'substances' or 'drugs' to cover any psychoactive substances whether legal or not. From a scientific perspective we need in the first instance to identify what a psychoactive substance is and what its effects are within the context it is used. This is a difficult area, precisely because individuals may experience the same drugs differently, and ideas of social acceptability change over time; however, it is important not only that policy is informed by science, but also that science accepts its moral obligations to society. This is a difficult area despite the efforts of governments to have evidence based policies (see Pawson, 2006) because science and policy are determined by quite different reinforcing events. For example, Hill and Newlin (2002: 375–9) argue that scientific development particularly in the field of evolution has caused controversy because of misuse of a biological explanation revolving around genetic determinism as a basis for eugenics, racism or sexism.

Within the European and American context from the nineteenth century onwards the involvement of Protestant evangelical Christianity has featured very strongly in dealing with one drug, namely 'the demon drink'. Worldwide the main provider of services for people with alcohol problems is Alcoholics Anonymous (AA) which has arisen out of a fusion of this form of Christianity and a medical view of addiction. This had developed, reinforced and maintained the disease concept of addiction, which in professional circles was in the ascendancy until the 1970s, and is still the approach taken by AA and other Twelve Step Fellowships. The arguments about whether addiction is best seen as a disease, or as a psychological or a social problem have occupied the minds of many academics and researchers, usually working within their own intellectual gulags. As Chapter 3 will show these debates are important because the definition you use may well inform the services that you recommend or provide and the way in which you deal with your own problems.

The use of language and labels is important, particularly in helping and therapeutic relationships because words can build up or destroy; in motivational interviewing, for example, one of the key tenets is that labelling such as getting someone to accept the label 'alcoholic' or 'addict' is not important and may be counter-productive (see Miller and Rollnick, 2002). Labels such as 'drug taking', 'substance abuse', 'addiction', 'substance misuse', 'addiction', and 'dependency' tend to be used interchangeably. 'Substance abuse' is a term that tends to be used in the USA, with the less pejorative 'substance misuse' being used in the UK.

Within this book the following definitions used by the Advisory Council on the Misuse of Drugs (ACMD) (2006) will be utilised:

- The term 'drugs' refers to all psychoactive substances which are used to alter thoughts, feelings and actions. These include those which can be legally sold, purchased or possessed (often with restrictions), and those which are illegal under the Misuse of Drugs Act (1971) in the UK, or the equivalent legislation in other jurisdictions.
- Drug use or substance use is drug taking in the form of ingestion through smoking, drinking or swallowing.
- Drug misuse or substance misuse is drug taking judged to be inappropriate or dangerous.
- Drug addiction or dependence is characterised by strong compulsions to take a drug/s and difficulty in stopping despite harmful consequences.

The ACMD has also developed the idea of hazardous use, which is use that has the capacity to cause harm, and also problem drug use which is defined as 'anyone who experiences social, physical, legal or psychological problems with one or more drugs (2006: 15). This definition recognises the wide range of problems that can result from drug use, and reflects is dimensional nature.

Personal responsibility and anti-discriminatory practice

Not everybody who uses a substance (legal or illegal) becomes addicted or necessarily experiences negative consequences or causes social harm. For those who do experience addiction the understanding of this from within the broad framework of biology, psychology and sociology and their disciplinary variants has led to a plethora of different models (these are reviewed by West (2001)). But at the heart of the debate concerning the nature of addiction and social responses to it is the argument about the degree to which an individual can be held responsible for their actions. There is a consensus that addiction is 'a behaviour over which an individual has impaired control, with harmful consequences' (Cottler (1993) and Rounsaville et al. (1993) cited in West (2001: 3–13)). For West (2006) this means that addiction needs to be categorised as a psychiatric disorder which in practice is not straightforward, and this will be discussed in some detail. However, the idea of impaired control, in the sense of someone who might not be able to stop doing something even though they want to, despite severe and lasting consequences, may help us to be more understanding and tolerant of people who are experiencing these problems. Any language or labels used should reflect an anti-discriminatory position.

The research agenda is fundamental to the process of finding the most effective and ethically based ways of helping people to overcome these difficulties, although Thom (1999) has observed that there is something like a ten-year time lag before research informs the policy or practice agenda. The aim of this book is not to go through these theories but to present the main models that are used in practice in dealing with addiction. The outline of the book is as follows:

Chapter 1 will review the profile of people presenting to health, social and support services and the prevalence of physical health, psychological and social problems. Reference will be made to the comparative literature in consideration of poly drug use (including alcohol and prescription drugs), mental health problems, physical health problems, offending behaviour, housing problems, unemployment and relationship difficulties. There will be a discussion of these various issues and the major theoretical explanations for the links between substance misuse and the various problem areas. This will lay the ground for the ensuing chapters.

Chapter 2 is concerned with the policy context and legal framework for the control of drugs. The major international treaties that govern the control of illicit drugs, and the UK's domestic legislation particularly the Misuse of Drugs Act (1971), will be reviewed. The chapter will consider the idea of relative harm that lies behind the concept of differential prohibition, and recent critiques of that approach given that neither alcohol nor tobacco is included in the legislation. New Labour's National Drug Strategy will be reviewed, as will the Licensing Act (2003) and the Alcohol Harm Reduction Strategy. Particular reference will be made to the perceived links between drug use and social exclusion with a review of policies related to New Labour's social inclusion agenda such as National Service Frameworks for health, mental health and social services, housing policy (particularly the Supporting People initiative), the policy response to dual diagnosis and developments in the National Probation Service.

Chapter 3 will discuss the development of the disease theory which was dominant in professional and self-help circles for most of the twentieth century. Its origins are complex, but these led to a fundamental shift in attitudes to people with alcohol problems and to the development of services to try and help those people. The strengths and limitations of this approach will be analysed, and its development into the Alcohol Dependence Syndrome (ADS) which was adopted by the World Health Organisation in 1977. As will be seen ADS was an important step in recognising alcohol dependence as being dimensional in nature as opposed to a unitary disease phenomenon, and thus opened up new perspectives in understanding and responding to alcohol related problems. In addition, the concept of a dependence syndrome became a key tool of analysis for other drugs as well.

Chapter 4 will consider the impact that the notion of drug use as a syndrome has had upon the public health agenda, in terms of prevention and working with specific problems. The importance of social policy as an instrument of public health will be discussed, along with the development of educative and advertising campaigns and harm minimisation approaches such as needle exchanges and substitute prescribing.

Chapter 5 will discuss the psychological revolution in the understanding and amelioration of addiction. Particular reference will be made to the developments in cognitive and behavioural approaches to understanding addiction. It will consider the impact of ideas that informed harm minimisation and controlled drinking approaches and the development of social learning techniques. Critical attention will be paid to the Transtheoretical Model of Change which has become ubiquitous in professional practice and encapsulates some core psychological constructs; these constructs, namely motivation, self-efficacy and self-esteem, will be examined.

Chapter 6 will review the contribution that neurobiology has made to our understanding of addiction, particularly in the light of the genetic revolution and our increased understanding of evolutionary processes.

Chapter 7 will review the main interventions in working with addiction, including self-help and Twelve Step Facilitation, cognitive behavioural approaches and motivational approaches. The evidence seems to suggest that all interventions have equivocal outcomes and that the most important factors are the interpersonal characteristics of the people running the interventions. There will be a discussion of empathy and motivational working as a statement of values in action.

Chapter 8 will review the notion of addiction as an example of a complex self-organising system. This idea arises from the application of complexity theory to human behaviour and reflects an approach that challenges linear approaches to understanding and working with addiction. This chapter will argue that this approach represents an important development in understanding the often paradoxical and counter-intuitive effects of addiction. Using a simple method called Cellular Automata (CA) it is possible to begin to model how complex systems emerge based upon the interaction of their component parts. This chapter will demonstrate CA as a basis for non-linear thinking and to argue that in working with a complex system, such as addiction, different approaches are required. Particular reference will be made to the evolutionary, dynamic and adaptive nature of the problems involved and the implications for service development. The shortcomings of using punitive and coercive approaches to working with addiction will be discussed.

Through the use of an extended case study, Chapter 9 will draw together the main themes of the book and encourage the reader to reflect upon the complex nature of the biopsychosocial paradigm, its component parts, and the ways in which problems can be overcome.

Throughout the text important points will be highlighted and issues for further discussion will be raised. Where possible, further useful reading or other resources will be indicated and links will be made between different sections of the book.

1

Drugs and Drug Users in Context

The aims of this chapter are to:

- define what a 'drug' is
- outline the major licit and illicit drugs along with their effects
- use comparative data to outline the prevalence of drug use
- use comparative data to establish the profile of people in terms of their drug use and the range of issues that they commonly present to specialist agencies as well as health, social welfare and law and order organisations.

In fact and fiction the history of humanity is replete with what Davenport-Hines (2001; 2004) has called the 'pursuit of oblivion'. In fiction Robert Graves (1992: 9) talks about the drunken God Dionysus and his followers the Maenads and the Centaurs, who washed down copious amounts of hallucinogenic mushrooms with wine and ivy ale thus inducing 'hallucinations, senseless rioting (involving running around the countryside tearing animals or children in pieces) prophetic insight, erotic energy and remarkable physical strength'. The use of psychoactive substances is a key feature in religious ceremonies from the Jewish Shabbat to the Christian Eucharist, and where alcohol has been proscribed, for example in Islamic countries, then coffee houses and the smoking of tobacco have assumed significance (Weinberg and Bealer, 2001). Conan Doyle's Sherlock Holmes is a frequenter of opium dens, and there is evidence to suggest that some of the most significant leaders in history, such as Alexander the Great (see Liappas et al., 2003), Stalin (see Sebag-Montefiori, 2002) and Churchill (Storr, 2008) (who was also never seen in public without a Havana cigar), had alcohol problems.

Although there has been the presence of psychoactive drugs in virtually all human cultures it has been the development of the industrial state over the last 300 years, and its commensurate colonial expansion (Gately 2001), that have given rise to the concern with addiction and drug related problems. Drug epidemics are nothing new, and we can consider two that were separated by 250 years. The gin epidemics of the eighteenth century and the heroin epidemics of the 1980s are strikingly similar, in that the contributing factors included urban poverty and the technology to mass produce the drugs and thus to improve the route of entry into the body. The invention of the distilling process to produce spirits allows higher concentrations of alcohol to be consumed and faster, so making drunkenness easier and more likely. Likewise the development of the hypodermic syringe allows heroin to enter into the bloodstream more rapidly for a quicker and bigger 'hit'. During the 1980s heroin use was found to be 'widespread' amongst predominantly socially excluded young people in cities and nearby towns, with estimated numbers between 100 and 150,000 users (Parker, 2005). Within the context of economic decline, and the lack of funding available to health and social services, heroin use had a major impact upon already disadvantaged communities. But compare these numbers with the gin epidemics. The eighteenth century was an age of prodigious drinking with the year 1750 seeing six million people (including children) drink 11 million gallons of gin (Heather and Robertson, 1997). Within the current context of concerns over the increasing consumption of alcohol within western industrialised societies, the situation is not seen as a drug epidemic in the same ways that increasing heroin use was and is seen to be. This is because of the social acceptability of alcohol and the part that it plays in our cultural and social life.

> Should we see alcohol as just another drug?

What is a drug?

> Take a few moments to jot down what you think a drug is, what drugs you use, what you see as the pleasurable and not so pleasurable consequences of that use, and any experiences you have of trying to change that use.

Goldstein (2001: 4) argues that:

> A drug is any chemical agent that affects biologic function … A psychoactive drug is one that acts in the brain to alter mood, thought processes or behaviour.

Nothing about drugs as such, even psychoactive ones, makes people like them or try to secure them. On the contrary when physicians prescribe drugs a major difficulty is getting patients to take them regularly … this 'compliance problem' is just as troublesome with many psychoactive drugs (such as those used to treat mental illness) as it is with drugs of other kinds.

We all use drugs of one kind or another usually because we have an expectation of the effects of those drugs, whether it is to get high, to relax, or to find some energy. This psychological expectation plays an important role in combination with the biological effects and crucially the social and environmental context as well. We can say that drugs act on the basis of a combination of physical effects on the brain and body, the psychological expectation that the individual has of the effects of the drug, as well as the influence of the peer group and social norms of the individual.

For a drug to work it has to be ingested (see below for different routes of entry to the body). The human brain then sends signals across nerve tracts via a system of chemical messengers which are called neurotransmitters, and which Goldstein (2001) refers to as the brain's own drugs. Different psycho-active drugs have their own ways of working with these neurotransmitters and can act on the nerve pathways as a mimic of those natural drugs, or to selectively block the activity of the natural drugs, or to enhance the natural action of a neurotransmitter.

The neurotransmitters are described as a kind of 'chemical key' which fits into designated 'keyholes' which are essentially receptor sites found on the surface of nerve cells. The psychoactive drug may be able to key into and unlock one or more kinds of receptor site and thus have its effect. The role of the brain and its evolutionary development will be discussed in detail in Chapter 6, but at this stage we need to know that particular neurotransmitters are implicated in a reward system that regulates behaviour such as eating, sex and drugs. (The neurobiology of drug use will be discussed in detail in Chapter 6.)

Drug classification

Usually drugs are classified according to the major mode of impact that they have on the mind (Edwards, 2004) and thus the following classifications are used by academics and practitioners:

- sedatives
- stimulants
- opiates

- hallucinogens
- mixed effects
- volatiles.

You will see from Table 1.1 that there are both immediate and longer term effects from using drugs (the table is not intended as a definitive guide to all problems experienced) and it is usually the desired immediate effect that is the reason for taking the drug. For example, someone attending a rave might use amphetamines or ecstasy to keep dancing all night, whereas a person wanting to relax may use alcohol or cannabis. However, none of these categories are clearly delineated in the sense that the effects of a particular drug will be mediated by the biology of the individual, the environment in which the drug is used (including other people in attendance), and the expectations that the individual has of the effects of that drug. In addition, of course, people may use a combination of drugs (poly drug use), at the same time, for differing effects. At this stage we are only considering the biological and psychological effects of some drugs. Issues of social control (in the form of legal sanctions based upon notions of relative harms) have not been raised, but will be discussed further in Chapter 2, and neither have the social consequences of drug use, which we will come to later in this chapter.

The worldwide prevalence of drugs

The United Nations Office of Drugs and Crime Prevention produced a World Drug Report (UNODC, 2006). The UNODC estimates that 200 million people worldwide (out of a population of 6,389 million) (4.9% of the population between the ages of 15 and 64) use illicit drugs. Of these 3.9% use cannabis, 0.5% amphetamines, 0.4% opiates, 0.2% ecstasy, 0.4% opiates (of which heroin is 0.3%) and cocaine 0.30%. Within this total population it is estimated that 25 million people (ages 15-64) are involved in problem drug use.

Adult drug use in the UK

In the UK the European Monitoring Centre for Drugs and Drug Addiction (EMCDDA) (2006), utilising the figures from the British Crime Survey (BCS) to monitor drug use, estimates that approximately one third of the adult population between the ages of 16 and 64 acknowledge having used some kind of illicit drug during their lifetime. People under the age of 35 are far more likely to use illicit drugs, with prevalence of use highest for those under 25 years of age. There is evidence to suggest that the

TABLE 1.1   *Drugs and their effects*

Name	Method of ingestion	Immediate effects	Longer term effects
Sedatives			
Barbiturates	Oral	Calmness/muscular relaxation/sleep. Large doses cause unconsciousness and death. Prescribed for anxiety, sleeplessness and sedation.	Physical dependence/ tolerance. Withdrawal symptoms such as anxiety, insomnia, irritability, convulsions, hallucinations and vomiting.
Benzodiazepines	Oral	As for barbiturates overdose but less lethal. Prescribed for anxiety and sedation. Combined with alcohol produces respiratory depression and impaired motor visual performance.	As for barbiturates.
Alcohol	Oral	Low dose can act as a stimulant but becomes a depressant as dose increases. Precise behavioural effects influenced by cognitive and social factors. Impairs judgement, visual motor performance, memory and concentration.	Heavy prolonged use leads to anxiety, depression, memory loss and physical illness. Liver damage and affects all major organs. Patterns of tolerance and dependence depend upon amount, pattern and extent of ingestion. Severe withdrawal symptoms include vomiting, sweating, hallucinations, convulsions and possibly death.
Stimulants			
Amphetamines	Oral or injection	User feels energetic, sometimes euphoric, and capable of prolonged concentration. At higher doses causes restlessness, irritability and aggression.	Psychosis, impulsive violence, depression. Suppression of appetite can cause malnutrition. Risk of hepatitis/HIV infection through sharing needles.
Cocaine	Snorting/eating or injecting	Euphoria, increased energy, enhanced mental alertness. Increased blood pressure, respiration and body temperature.	Restlessness, insomnia, paranoia, psychosis.

TABLE 1.1   *(Continued)*

Name	Method of ingestion	Immediate effects	Longer term effects
Caffeine	Tea, coffee, soft drinks or chocolate	Delays onset of sleep. Increased performance at simple intellectual tasks.	Insomnia, anxiety and depression. Withdrawal symptoms such as headache and irritability.
Opiates			
Opiate narcotics (includes opium, heroin and methadone)	Oral, smoking or injection	Brief stimulation of the brain then depression of the central nervous system. Feelings of euphoria, possible restlessness, nausea and vomiting. At higher doses respiratory failure and possibly death.	Tolerance develops to many of the desired effects. Withdrawal symptoms may include cramps, sweats and diarrhoea. Risk of HIV/hepatitis infection through shared needles.
Hallucinogens			
Mescaline	Eating or injection	Increased behavioural activity and hallucinations. Increased blood pressure, pulse and body temperature.	Psychotic reaction and unpredictable flashbacks of the original experience.
Datura (magic mushrooms)	Eating	As for mescaline.	As for mescaline.
Lysergic acid diethylamide (LSD)	Oral, snorting or injection	Changes perception, thought and mood. Hallucinations.	Flashbacks and psychosis.
Volatiles			
Solvents	Sniffing	Euphoria and excitement. Muscular unco-ordination and depressed reflexes.	Weight loss, nosebleeds, kidney, liver and brain damage.
Drugs with mixed effects			
Ecstasy	Oral or injection	Altered perception, pleasant feelings, stimulation, hallucinations, vomiting and agitation.	Not yet known.
Cannabis	Smoking or eating	Euphoria, sedation and impairment of short term memory and psychomotor skills. Large doses cause hallucinations, delusions and anxiety	Loss of energy, impaired memory and concentration and respiratory disorders through smoking.
Nicotine	Smoking, chewing or snorting (snuff)	Stimulation of central nervous system. Increased heart rate and respiration. Used *for* relaxation and avoidance of withdrawal.	Cancers (particularly of the lung), respiratory disease, restlessness and anxiety.

Source: adapted from Edwards, 2004; Barber, 1995

prevalence of use and particularly first time use is declining. Males are more likely to report drug use than females, with those differences tending to become more significant with age. The EMCDDA argues that in 2005/6 based upon the results of 29,631 respondents cannabis was the most widely used illicit drug across all age groups at 8.7%, which was very close to the figure of 10.5% for any drug used. All other drug use was much lower with cocaine at 2.4%, ecstasy at 1.6%, amphetamines at 1.3%, magic mushrooms at 1%, LSD at 0.3% and crack at 0.2%. Opiate use is not included in these figures but the EMCCDA estimates the prevalence of opioid use at a national level to range roughly between one and six cases per 1,000 population aged 15–64.

Poly drug use

Evidence from major studies across the developed world indicates that poly drug use is the norm for many people, and not necessarily those who have a dependency problem. For example, there is an acceptance that a key feature of the club and dance scene is young people experimenting with a variety of substances (Parker et al., 1998). However, within the literature there is disagreement over what the term 'poly drug use' should actually entail in terms of substances (whether legal or illegal) and the timings of their ingestion (Hunt, 2007). Studies such as the National Treatment Outcome Study and the Drug and Alcohol Outcome Treatment Study (see below) show that within the 'clinical' population this is a major issue in relation to detoxification and rehabilitation.

The European School Survey Project on Alcohol and Other Drugs (ESPAD) (see www.espad.org) was set up in 1994 to study adolescent substance use in Europe from a comparative and longitudinal perspective. Four data collections have taken place from the participating countries in 1995, 1999, 2003 and 2007, with new countries joining for each survey point.

The ESPAD findings clearly demonstrate a strong emphasis on poly drug use amongst those people turning 16 years of age in the year that the data are collected. In the UK the drinking of alcohol by adolescents and drunkenness are above the average for the ESPAD countries as a whole, and have stayed relatively stable since 1995. In 1995 90% of adolescents had consumed alcohol in the last 12 months, and 91% in 1999 and 2003 respectively. This compares to the ESPAD average of 80% for 1995, 82% for 1999, and 81% for 2003. Of even more concern are the figures for drunkenness over the same period, with the UK figures being 70%, 69% and 68% for the respective years as compared to the ESPAD averages of

47%, 51% and 50%. Although alcohol consumption has remained much the same over the same period the use of alcohol and pills in combination has declined from 20% to the ESPAD average of 7%.

By 2003 cigarette smoking amongst adolescents in the UK had fallen below the ESPAD average of 63% to 58%, and also tranquiliser and sedative use standing at 2% as compared to the ESPAD average of 7%. In addition, the use of inhalants which was at 20% in 1995 (compared to the ESPAD average of 9%) had dropped to 12 % in 1995, slightly below the ESPAD average of 10%. However, any drug but cannabis stood at 9% compared to the ESPAD average of 6% and cannabis use was at 38% as compared to the 20% ESPAD average.

The early and increased use of combinations of substances are important factors in the increased risk, not only of drug dependency (Li et al., 2007b) but also of the concurrence of mental health problems (see Chapter 5), as well as the associated problems of poverty and social exclusion.

The UNODC (2006) argues that the demand for drug treatment tends to mirror the availability of particular drugs, with the exception of cannabis. Given the extent of cannabis use across the world only a small proportion of users will seek treatment, although this number is growing in line with use. In Africa most treatment sought is for cannabis, in Asia and Europe it is for opiates, and in South America for cocaine. For the use of amphetamines treatment demand is highest in Asia followed by Oceania, North America, Europe, and Africa.

The social context of substance misuse in the UK

The UK Government (Home Office, 2002) estimated that there are 250,000 Class A drug users (see Chapter 2 for the system of classification) who account for 99% of the costs of drug misuse in England and Wales. The National Drug Strategy (Home Office 1998; 2002) was largely based on the National Treatment Outcome Research Study (NTORS) (see Gossop et al., 2003). NTORS was the first large scale, prospective and multi-site treatment outcome study of substance misusers carried out in the UK. It provides a useful source of information about the problems that service users arrive at treatment with, the operational characteristics of the programmes themselves, and the outcomes from those programmes. A sample of 1075 people was established from 54 different agencies (Drug Dependency Units, Rehabilitation Centres, and Methadone Maintenance and Methadone Reduction programmes). Of particular concern to New Labour was the perceived link between drug use and crime, and mainly acquisitive crime.

NTORS researched four problem domains including substance use, health risk behaviour, physical psychological health and personal/social functioning. Since that study was started in 1995, and with the implementation of the National Drug Strategy changing the context of drug service provision (particularly with the expansion of criminal justice interventions) combined with changing patterns of drug use, the Drug Treatment Outcomes Research Study (DTORS) has been developed (Jones et al., 2007). DTORS is to run for three years following 1,796 adults through treatment and is researching similar problem domains to NTORS.

Age, ethnicity and gender

The baseline information at intake shows that the gender and age profile for DTORS was 73% male and 27% female, with 20% being between 16 and 24 years of age, 45% at 25 to 34 years of age, 27% at 35 to 44 years of age, and 7% at 45 years and over. Of these 89% were White in terms of their ethnicity, 4% of mixed ethnicity, 3% Black, 3% Asian, and 2% 'Other' including Chinese. Those people with crack as their main problem were more likely to be Black, with heroin the main drug for White treatment seekers.

Family context

The partners of 38% of those seeking treatment also used drugs and women were more likely to have a drug using partner. About half of the cohort had children under 16, but only about 25% lived with their children. That problematic drug use has the potential to impact negatively upon children and families has become an increasing concern for policy makers as well as practitioners, with over a million children in the UK having parents with substance misuse problems (Forrester et al., 2008). Within the UK 'Every Child Matters' (www.dcsf.gov.uk/everychildmatters) is the key government policy to ensure that all areas of government are working together in addressing the needs of children; this includes in working with substance use and misuse. The Advisory Council on the Misuse of Drugs (2003, cited in Barnard and McKeganey, 2004) estimated that 2-3% of all children under the age of 16 have parents with drug problems.

In their review of the published research (which has come mainly from America) looking into the impact of parental drug use on children, Barnard and McKeganey (2004) identified three key areas:

1   The impact on the home environment and child care.
2   Parent–child relationships.
3   Child behaviour.

Due to the relapsing nature of addiction (see Chapter 3) followed by periods of recovery and then relapse, household stability can vary. This means that when a parent is increasingly involved in drug use then child care and the home can become secondary considerations. This can then lead to a lack of care towards the child in the form of food, clothing and hygiene, and put the child substantially at risk of harm. Barnard and McKeganey (2004) cite a study by Shulman, Shapira and Hirschfield (2000) which showed that 83% ($n=100$) of assessed children of parents attending methadone clinics in New York had medical or nutritional disorders of varying degrees. Studies in the USA have shown that it is neglect rather than physical or sexual abuse that is the main reason for social workers to intervene with drug using parents and also the main reason for children to be taken into care.

Barnard and McKeganey's review demonstrates as well that a preoccupation with drug use is likely to impair a parent's ability to be warm, consistent and emotionally responsive to a child's needs. The children of drug using parents are also more likely to be separated from their families, and there would appear to be an increasing negative relationship between the severity of the drug problem and the quality of relationship. In particular increasing drug involvement was significantly associated with less supervision of the child, a more punitive approach to discipline, and disagreements between partners over disciplinary issues and less positive involvement with the child.

As a consequence of these levels of deprivation then there is an increased likelihood of problematic patterns of behaviour by children of drug dependent parents. Studies reviewed demonstrate heightened levels of anxiety and depression amongst these groups of children, as well as hyperactivity, impulsivity and aggression and behaviours consonant with attention deficit hyperactivity disorder.

These issues have the potential to lead to other problems for the individuals and the communities in which they live, one of which is the potential for children themselves to develop drug problems as they grow up. This debate concerning nature versus nurture is a complex one, and will be discussed in Chapter 6 when we look at the importance of genetic influences on addiction. However, a systematic review by Beckett et al. (2004) of studies into an understanding of problem drug use amongst young people argued that poor parental control is possibly the main determinant of the level of problematic drug use due to the internalisation of parental attitudes to drug use.

A study by Forrester et al. (2008) evaluated a programme called 'Option 2' which was commissioned by the Welsh Assembly Government to work with families of parents with substance misuse problems. The aims of the programme were to safeguard children at risk of harm, to improve family functioning, and to reduce the need for the children to be taken into care. The intervention is short and intensive, lasting between four to six weeks, but with a social worker available 24 hours a day and with workers utilising motivational and solution focused approaches. Parents felt that they got a better service from Option 2 in comparison with social services, and were appreciative of the excellent listening and communication skills of the workers, and their commitment to and knowledge of the family situation. The result was that, by the end of 2006, 24% of Option 2 children were still in care as opposed to 33% of children not using this service, and 68% were still living at home from the Option 2 group in comparison to 56% of the others.

This study found that, with the families with fewer and less complex problems, these changes were lasting, but for more complex issues the problems resurfaced once the Option 2 support had been withdrawn. This research demonstrates a number of key issues, including the importance of motivational working (see Chapter 7) and of concurrent, continuous and aftercare services (see Chapters 8 and 9).

Accommodation

DTORS shows that 40% of dependent drug users were living in unstable accommodation which is very similar to the previous NTORS findings of 7% rough sleepers, 5% living in squats, 8% in temporary hostel accommodation, and 17% in more than one type of accommodation.

An assessment of the international literature on effective substance misuse services for homeless people was conducted by Pleace (2008) on behalf of the Scottish Government. There is evidence that substance misuse amongst rough sleeping young people is at a higher rate than in the general population. Pleace found that the relationship between substance misuse and homelessness is complex and mutually reinforcing, with becoming homeless leading to an increased risk of substance misuse, and substance misuse leading to an increased risk of homelessness. As will be seen when we discuss complexity theory (see Chapter 8), these interaction effects are crucial to our understanding of the ways in which a system of addiction is perpetuated. In addition, Pleace found a strong correlation between mental health problems, substance misuse and homelessness, with similar patterns across the European Union, North America and Japan (see Chapter 5 for a discussion on dual diagnosis). There is a recognition amongst practitioners and policy makers that 'Appropriate and sustainable housing is a foundation for successful rehabilitation of drug users…[and] is crucial [in] sustaining employment [and] drug treatment.' (Office of the Deputy Prime Minister, 2004: 2).

Education and employment

The DTORS research shows that 38% had left school before 16 and 77% reported being unemployed, with NTORS demonstrating that 28% were self-supporting with a wage or casual work and 12% had a job. In their review of the literature McSweeney and Hough (2006) found again that there are mutually reinforcing and complex barriers to drug users accessing the labour market. These include the following:

- limited academic qualifications and work experience
- poor literacy skills coupled with dyslexia
- skills and training deficits coupled with low confidence, self-esteem and motivation
- poor job seeking skills
- relationship problems and fractured social networks
- criminal records and employer attitudes
- only offered temporary, low paid jobs
- mental health problems.

These issues were also often coupled with high levels of temporary or inadequate accommodation.

Health issues and treatment contact

Given this evidence for multiple interacting and mutually reinforcing problems and needs it is not surprising that 23% of the DTORS cohort had a mental health diagnosis, with 43% having had lifetime contact with mental health services. This will be discussed in detail, but at this stage we need to acknowledge that if you have a drug and/or alcohol problem you are far more likely to have a mental health problem and vice versa. In the NTORS cohort feelings of hopelessness were experienced by 62%, terror and panic 41%, suicidal thoughts 29%, chest pains 38%, sleep disturbance 81%, weight loss 68%, and dental problems 54%.

Drug use

In the four weeks prior to interview 62% reported using heroin, 44% crack, 25% benzodiazepines, and 50% alcohol. Injecting drug use was reported by 37% and 48% of injectors admitted to sharing equipment in the previous four weeks. Of the opiate users 76% reported poly drug use in combinations with other opiates, benzodiazepines or alcohol. Thirty-seven per cent reported poly drug use in combination with injecting and 9% reported overdosing in the previous three months.

Criminal activity

DTORS showed that over 39% had committed acquisitive crime in the four weeks prior to interview and 22% reported offending to support a drug habit, with 18% reporting that they had offended under the influence of drugs. Of all the people interviewed on DTORS, whether they were referred through the criminal justice system or not, 73% reported having committed a crime in the previous 12 months. This would seem to support the basis of the National Drug Strategy (Home Office, 1998; 2002) of a substantial link between drug use and crime. However non-criminal justice referrals reported their proceeds from crime over the previous four weeks at an average of £130, with criminal justice referrals at an average of £200, which would seem to indicate relatively low levels of crime. The crimes in order of frequency in NTORS are shoplifting 38%, selling drugs 29%, fraud 15%, burglary 12%, robbery 5%, and other theft 5%. A key feature of the National Drugs Strategy (Home Office, 1998; 2002) has been the expansion of criminal justice interventions to address particularly the relationship between drug use and acquisitive crime (see Chapter 2).

This expansion in criminal justice activity can be seen by the fact that 55% of the DTORS cohort receiving treatment were subject to a court mandated Drug Rehabilitation Requirement. The referrals that came via the criminal justice system had more complex offending patterns, were more likely to be using crack, more likely to be in unstable accommodation, more likely to be separated from their children and more likely to be from black and minority ethnic communities. In addition 71% of all referrals had previously had structured day or residential treatment, and likewise in research on drug use amongst newly sentenced prisoners Stewart (2009) found 51% had had previous treatment in the community and 17% in a previous prison term. This not only supports the relapsing nature of addiction (see Chapters 3,5,6 and 7) but also in the case of prison demonstrates that despite most prisoners entering custody (either sentenced or on remand) with a history of drug and alcohol misuse, many have not previously received any help with their problems (Social Exclusion Unit, 2002).

The findings from NTORS and DTORS are broadly in line with other longitudinal studies carried out in Ireland, Australia and the USA (see further resources). The key issues arising from these studies are the importance of the multiple interacting needs that individuals experience in relation to their substance use, and the ways in which agencies respond and try to address those needs.

Alcohol

The two studies also demonstrate that alcohol is a major issue which is not only implicated in the risk of drug overdose (see Chapter 4), but was also something that NTORS found was not being addressed in drug treatment centres. NTORS show major improvements across all of the problem domains with the exception of alcohol consumption. This may reflect the acceptability and availability of alcohol as a legal substance, and one which drug treatment centres had not thought was their primary concern. This problem is also not reflected in funding mechanisms for organisations which have very different budgets for alcohol and illicit drugs.

The figures for illicit drug use stand in stark contrast to those for alcohol, with the estimate that (at 2003 figures) 90% of the world population have exposure to alcohol (Rehm et al., 2003). Illicit drug use also stands in contrast to the estimated 28% of the world adult population using tobacco (UNODC, 2006). Despite this disparity in the numbers using alcohol and those using illicit drugs, there is far more of a concerted focus on dealing with the latter, from the International Conventions of the United Nations through to domestic legislations (see Chapter 2).

The statistics on world alcohol consumption and drinking patterns have been reviewed by Babor et al. (2003) and show some interesting features. Firstly that across all areas there are more male drinkers than female drinkers, but also that the level of alcohol dependence within a population is directly correlated with the total consumption of alcohol per person. For example, in the World Health Organisation (WHO) designation of the 'Americas' (USA, Canada and Cuba) the total consumption (measured in litres of absolute alcohol per person aged 15 years and over per year) is 9.3 litres, with a rate of alcohol dependence standing at 5.1%. Likewise in the parts of Europe that are constituted by Germany, France and the UK the total consumption is 12.9 litres per person, with an alcohol dependence rate of 3.4%. When these figures are compared with areas that are largely made up of Islamic countries where alcohol is largely proscribed we find, for example, that in areas that contain Iran and Saudi Arabia the total consumption is 1.3 litres per person, and for Afghanistan and Pakistan 0.6 litres, with both regions having alcohol dependence rates of 0%.

This relationship between the amount of alcohol consumed and the increased risk of problems is a significant issue, and is not one that for example the UK Government has accepted in its review of the licensing laws (see Chapter 2). It will also be discussed further in relation to disease and ADS in Chapter 3.

Safe levels of drinking

In the UK, because alcohol is a legal commodity, notions of harmful use are judged against the guidelines that are given by the Department of Health on safe drinking, which in turn are predicated upon the measurement of units. One unit equals a standard measure of one standard strength drink (half a pint of beer, a glass of wine, a single spirit, etc.) and the NHS recommends that men drink no more than three or four units per day and women no more than two or three.

Binge drinking

Binge drinking is defined as drinking eight or more units of alcohol in one session if you are a man, and more than six units in one session if you are a woman. There is evidence to suggest that binge drinking can be far more harmful both physically and mentally than slow steady drinking.

Adult alcohol use in the UK

In 2004 the Alcohol Needs Assessment Research Project (ANARP) conducted the first national alcohol needs assessment in England (Department of Health, 2004). This survey found that between the ages of 16-64, 38% of men and 16% of women have an Alcohol Use Disorder (AUD) (ranging between problems and dependence, see the discussion on ADS in Chapter 3). This equates to 8.2 million people, or just over one quarter of the population. Additionally, there are 1.1 million people nationally (6% of men and 2% of women) who are alcohol dependent, and there are 21% of men and 9% of women who are binge drinkers. The survey found that all AUDs decline with age and that black and minority ethnic groups have a lower prevalence of hazardous/harmful alcohol use, but a similar prevalence of alcohol dependence compared with the white population. Importantly the survey found that there are extremely low levels of formal identification, treatment and referral of patients with Alcohol Use Disorders by GPs and that there was a tendency to over identify younger patients with AUD compared with older patients. Of the patients who were identified by GPs as having an AUD and requiring specialist treatment (71%) many were not referred because of perceived difficulties in accessing services due to waiting lists, and patients choosing not to engage in specialist treatment. The consumption of alcohol at problematic levels has huge implications for personal health and health services. Gossop et al. (2007) carried out a review of the health problems amongst problem drinkers across six European cities and their findings can be seen in Table 1.2. It is interesting to note that alcohol use affects every part of the human organism and that 60% of problematic alcohol users require some kind of treatment.

TABLE 1.2   *Prevalence of health problems amongst drinkers*

Health domain	Disorder present	Moderate/severe disorder	Requires treatment
Cardiovascular	28%	11%	24%
Neurological	26%	11%	18%
Gastrointestinal and liver	48%	17%	28%
Respiratory	14%	6%	9%
Endocrine and metabolic	10%	5%	8%
Musculoskeletal	20%	8%	14%
Dermatological	10%	3%	9%
Dental	29%	12%	25%
Genitourinary	10%	2%	7%
Any health problem	79%	40%	60%

Source: Gossop et al., (2007) 'Physical health problems among patients seeking treatment for alchohol use disorders: a study in six European cities', *Addiction Biology*, 12(2): 190–6.

Multiple interacting needs

The issue of multiple needs has been and continues to be the major challenge for substance misuse, welfare and criminal justice agencies. Identifying what the individual's primary problem is, whether housing as opposed to drug use or mental health problems as opposed to withdrawal symptoms, raises real problems in responding to those needs through public services. This is because public services are usually funded to provide a specific service, for specific categories of people. The issue of 'dual diagnosis' will be discussed in Chapter 5, but this is an area where separate services have developed to address either substance misuse or mental health problems. For an individual who has both sets of problems concurrently the substance misuse service may ask them to resolve their mental health problem before working with them, and the mental health service wants the substance misuse problem resolved before they work with them. This is also an area that has been under-researched and under-theorised (with the possible exception of 'dual diagnosis' and working with survivors of childhood sexual misuse) despite presenting some of the most significant challenges to the provision of public services in terms of assessment and intervention.

In the academic and professional literature the concept of multiple needs is often described in multiple ways that reflect the theoretical, political and professional orientation of those doing the describing. Some of the labels used are: complex needs, poly problem individuals, crimino-genic need, distal needs, dual diagnosis, social exclusion, alcohol/drug related problems. There has been an important debate, notably instigated by Fiorentine (1998), as to whether within substance misuse treatment set-tings it is necessary to address other needs as well or whether the focus should be on the addiction. Fiorentine looks particularly at these 'distal needs' in relation to Post Traumatic Stress Disorder (PTSD) of which there is a high prevalence in treatment settings. He argues that the addressing of wider issues is largely a humanistic response, and particularly as needs may emerge during the course of treatment, with a good example being the disclosure of experiencing sexual abuse as a child. However, his evidence suggests that resolving abuse issues is not necessarily related to overcoming substance misuse issues.

CASE EXAMPLE

Kath is a 32-year-old woman, who has been referred by her General Practitioner for a residential detoxification from alcohol. Kath lives in a privately rented bedsit, and works night shifts in a factory. The scars on her arms indicate that she self-harms, she has medication to help her sleep, and she also take anti-depressants and smokes tobacco. Kath is invited to attend a six-week residential aftercare programme on completion of her detox and she declines, choosing to go back to her flat. Within one month she is admitted for another alcohol detox, and again declines the offer of aftercare. Within six months she is detoxed again and this time chooses aftercare, partly on the basis that she is being evicted from her flat, but she does not complete the programme. Within the next few months she is detoxed again and asks for aftercare, but this time disclosing that she was seriously sexually abused as a child by her grandfather. Kath then states that she has been seeing a Clinical Nurse Specialist for adult survivors of abuse, and asks for a three-way meeting between a member of staff from the aftercare programme, the Nurse Specialist, and herself. The meeting is held and a course of action is agreed in terms of assessing need and establishing a care plan.

In working through issues of disclosure with her nurse, Kath would start drinking again and/or self-harm, and she would experience significant nightmares (this is why she had worked night shifts). The Nurse Specialist would work with the disclosure, and the aftercare programme would address relapse prevention and relapse management techniques. It was a requirement of the programme that Kath remain abstinent, and so they had to find ways of managing her relapse situation, and getting her back onto the programme as quickly as pos-sible. During the work with Kath a shifting levels approach was used through the Transtheoretical Model of Change (see Chapter 5) which allowed for periods of stability to do more 'in depth' work on trauma, followed by relapse work and so forth. Over time the periods of relapse decreased and Kate was able to lead a more settled life.

When we consider the case of Kath is it possible to say that the issues of child-hood abuse, substance misuse, depression and self-harm are not all intrinsically linked?

If substance misuse, and particularly addiction, is seen within a biopsychosocial paradigm, then it is to be expected that problems will occur across all three areas and all of these will interact with each other. The example of Kath although described in a very superficial way is not untypical of people presenting to services with multiple needs, many of them apparently intractable. In an era of 'managed care', and perform-ance management within public services, these organisations are now focused more than ever on prioritising their work. Within the UK, for example, the National Probation Service will only work with needs that are 'criminogenic', that is those issues which are related to offending behaviour.

Conclusion

In the history of mankind, and indeed in the experience of our evolution-ary forebears (see Chapter 6), the use of psychoactive substances has been a constant feature of our human experience. Over the course of that time the types of drugs used have changed as they have moved in and out of social acceptability. All drug use whether legal or illegal carries the risk of harm which is mediated by biological, psychological and social circum-stances, but the use of a substance in itself, whether that is cocaine, heroin, alcohol or tobacco, is not necessarily problematic. The risks are escalated by the severity, duration, frequency and mode of ingestion, and one of the difficulties here is that because some drugs are illegal their use is seen as 'problematic', whereas some people may be using illicit substances but not experiencing any negative consequences, unless they are caught and con-victed of possessing and using drugs. The harms of drug use become a part of the overall problem as we will see in the following chapters, and this will ultimately lead us to a discussion concerning multi-agented systems and complexity theory (see Chapter 8).

Useful resources

Australian Treatment Outcome Research Study – www.ncbi.nlm.nih.gov/pubmed/
   17364836

Drug Treatment Outcome Research Study – www.dtors.org.uk

Drug and Alcohol Treatment Outcome Study (USA) – www.datos.org/

European Monitoring Centre on Drugs and Drug Addiction – www.emcdda.
   europa.eu/

Research Outcome Study (Ireland) – www.nacd.ie/activities/rosie.html

United Nations Office of Drugs and Crime – www.unodc.org/

2

The Policy Context and Legal Framework

The aims of this chapter are to:

- review the international, regional and domestic responses to drug use
- outline within the UK context the key policies related to the use of drugs and their effects
- compare and contrast alcohol and cannabis to explore the related themes of 'differential prohibition' and 'relative harmfulness', and their application to the classification of drugs.

For most countries there is a range of laws and policies that will impinge upon the control and supply of drugs. It is important that both the practitioner and the academic are familiar with these as drug use is a factor that all professions working within welfare and caring jobs will come across, and very often at an interface with law enforcement and criminal justice agencies. This wider matrix of problems gives rise to the necessity for interdisciplinary and multi-agency approaches which in turn raise a number of theoretical and practical issues.

The key focus for this chapter is the notion of 'relative harm' that lies behind the concept of 'differential' prohibition which in the UK is enshrined in the Misuse of Drugs Act (1971). This piece of legislation is based upon the major international conventions that define and control illicit drugs. The concept of relative harm will be used as a tool of analysis for the Licensing Act (2003) and the Alcohol Harm Reduction Strategy which constitute a major piece of drug legislation and policy. This approach which hitherto has not been applied to alcohol or nicotine has increasingly come under scrutiny due to its inconsistency (ACMD, 2006; House of Commons Science and Technology Committee, 2005/2006). In so doing the chapter will consider New Labour's National Drug Strategy with particular reference to the perceived links between drugs use, social exclusion and crime. This will include a review of policies related to New Labour's social inclusion agenda such as the National Service Frameworks for health, mental health and social services, housing policy, the policy response to dual diagnosis and developments in the National Probation Service.

As might be expected of the biopsychosocial nature of drug use and its related problems, a pragmatic, multi-agency and interdisciplinary set of responses has developed across time within the UK context. The implementation of Tackling Drugs Together (HM Government, 1995) which established Drug Action Teams as multi-agency cross cutting 'virtual' organisations, was a seminal moment in British drugs policy. This was a much needed impetus for a multi-agency approach which was then built upon by the incoming Labour Government in 1997 to deliver the National Drug Strategy (Home Office, 1998). However, despite the welcomed investment that went into providing improved drugs services, via the newly established National Treatment Agency for Substance Misuse, the strategy failed to address the issue of alcohol; this was despite the NTORS research clearly demonstrating that alcohol is a major factor in poly drug use and the reality that many providers of services were dealing with in addressing multiple needs (see Chapter 1).

This example nicely highlights some of the contradictions that policy agendas throw up, particularly when those policies and legislative procedures do not keep track with the evidence base. Despite the evidence base clearly demonstrating that people are presenting to services with multiple inter-relating problems, the policy response has taken a more focused single track approach.

Why are policy responses important?

Public policy or social policy is a 'term applied to a formal decision or a plan of action that has been taken by, or has involved, a state organisation'. (Richards and Smith, 2002: 1). Increasingly governments have sought policies that are evidence based, and in their search for solutions to social and economic problems have involved a wide range of technocrats and scientists in the formulation of these policies (see Chapter 8).

However, there is some debate as to whether scientific findings inform drugs policy (see House of Commons Science and Technology Committee, 2005/2006), even by the UK Government's own criteria for relative harm as laid out in the Misuse of Drugs Act (1971) (see below). This piece of legislation set up an Advisory Council on the Misuse of Drugs (ACMD), drawn from experts in the field, to inform the Home Secretary on drugs policy. However, the Science and Technology Committee's report found that very often decisions had been taken by government without consultation with the ACMD. Drugs are a highly politicised topic and one that is fraught with difficulty when trying to have the kind of rational public debate which should inform the development of policy in line with research findings. Most people who use caffeine, nicotine or alcohol do not see themselves as drug users and this is a major problem when talking about drugs, with the tendency to think only about illegal drugs. As is evident from the previous chapter, drug use in its broadest sense (that is whether legal or illegal) gives rise to a range of problems, and in reality some of those problems are caused by the legislative responses to the perceived problems caused by harmful drugs. For example, criminalising certain drug use may amplify the problems that socially excluded people are already experiencing. If a person has a criminal record because of their drug use then this can create problems in terms of maintaining interpersonal relationships, accessing housing, and finding employment.

As we will begin to discover the consumption of drugs (whether legal or not) is a dynamic issue, giving rise to variations in patterns of consumption and the benefits and costs associated with that use (Caulkins, 2007). This requires that the responses to those problems are as dynamic as the problems themselves. That is a tall order, but it does beg the question of what kind of legislation is required to respond to these issues. Should the legislation be framed as criminal law (as in the 1971 Act) or as part of a wider social policy agenda that is seen to be responsive to the needs of society, or is there a 'third way', which has been encapsulated by the so-called 'British System' (see below)?

Consider the following two statements as a clear example of the nature of the debate about drugs that exists at the highest levels within government both nationally and internationally:

> *Drugs are everywhere,* say alarmed parents. *The drug problem is out of control,* cries the media. *Legalize drugs to reduce crime,* say some commentators. Such exasperation is understandable in the many communities where illicit drugs cause crime, illness, violence and death. Yet worldwide statistical evidence points to a different reality: drug control is working and the world drug problem is being contained. (United Nations Office on Drugs and Crime, 2006: 1)

> In the course of our Inquiry it has become inescapably clear to us that the eradication of drug use is not achievable and is not therefore either a realistic or a sensible goal of public policy. (Runciman, 1999: 1)

Both of these bodies are concerned to 'control and limit the demand for and supply of illicit drugs' (Runciman, 1999: 1) but have very different views upon the effectiveness of the current approaches taken. The United Nations predominantly takes the view that it is possible to create a drug free world, in the sense of the continued prohibition of drugs of harm, through an enforcement, disruption and education agenda. As a consequence of this there is a system of global drug prohibition in place that is supervised by the United Nations (Levine, 2003), and particularly through the work of the International Narcotics Control Board. The three major drug control treaties brokered by the United Nations seek to enforce this prohibition (Fazey, 2003; Levine, 2003) by codifying international control measures so as to ensure the availability of narcotic drugs and psychotropic substances for medical and scientific purposes, and to prevent their diversion into illicit channels.

The legislative framework

Through the World Health Organisation the United Nations defines illicit drug use through the use of four levels of analysis (see unodc.org):

1 Any chemical entity or mixture of entities, the administration of which alters the biological function of the living organism.
2 The use to which the substance is put (this excludes legitimate medical use for the alleviation of disease).
3 A restriction to psychoactive drugs that alter mood, cognition and behaviour.
4 Drugs which are self-administered and impair health or social functioning.

The aim of this definition as enshrined within the conventions is to ensure that psychoactive substances are only cultivated and developed for proper medical and scientific use, and to ensure also that they are not diverted into illicit channels.

The United Nations conventions on illicit drugs

The Single Convention on Narcotic Drugs (1961)

The adoption of this Convention was regarded as a milestone in the history of international drug control. The Single Convention codified all existing multilateral treaties on drug control and extended the existing control systems to include the cultivation of plants that were grown as the raw materials of narcotic drugs. The principal objectives of the Convention are to limit the possession, use, trade in, distribution, import, export, manufacture and production of drugs exclusively to medical and scientific purposes and to address drug trafficking through international cooperation to deter and discourage drug traffickers. The Convention also established the International Narcotics Control Board, merging the Permanent Central Board and the Drug Supervisory Board (www.incb.org/incb/convention_1961.html).

Convention on Psychotropic Substances 1971

This Convention established an international control system for psychotropic substances. It responded to the diversification and expansion of the spectrum of drugs of abuse and introduced controls over a number of synthetic drugs according to their abuse potential on the one hand and their therapeutic value on the other (www.incb.org/incb/convention_1971.html).

United Nations Convention against the Illicit Traffic in Narcotic Drugs and Psychotropic Substances, 1988

This Convention provided comprehensive measures against drug trafficking, including provisions against money laundering and the diversion of precursor chemicals. It also provided for international cooperation through, for example, the extradition of drug traffickers, controlled deliveries and the transfer of proceedings (www.incb.org/incb/convention_1988.html).

The UK is a signatory to all of these conventions and is required to uphold the aims and objectives of each convention in its domestic law making. It is possible for signatories to these conventions to introduce stricter domestic legislation than that which is demanded by the conventions, but they cannot introduce more lenient approaches (Fazey, 2003). The Select Committee on Home Affairs (2002) notes that although this restricts unilateral action on the part of the UK when legislating on drug issues, there is possibly more room for manoeuvre than is usually acknowledged. The Committee argues that this is because 'the treaties do not lay down specific control mechanisms within the basic premise of criminality of drug possession and supply' (paragraph 266).

The Misuse of Drugs Act (1971)

Following on from these internationally agreed definitions the British government introduced the Misuse of Drugs Act (1971), which since its inception has remained the cornerstone of UK policy. The legislation is only concerned with drugs that are banned or only permissible for use in scientific and medical efforts and therefore, for instance, does not cover the use of alcohol or nicotine. This is an important point and we will return to it in due course.

> In your view should there be one piece of legislation to cover all drugs, including alcohol and tobacco, alongside all those which are currently illegal?

The purposes of the 1971 Act are to provide means for controlling all drugs and to divide these drugs into three classes in their descending degree of danger (A, B and C) and to grade the penalties for misusing drugs in each class accordingly. The Act distinguishes between unlawful possession and trafficking and creates new trafficking offences with severe punishments; continues to require the notification of drug addicts to the Home Office (this was a continued requirement of the Dangerous Drugs Act 1967) and restricts the prescription of drugs of dependence to them; allows for the provision of special treatment centres; and gives the Home Secretary powers to act quickly in the case of over-prescribing by general practitioners. It brings new substances under control and makes necessary regulations for the control of production, supply and possession of those substances; and allows for the demand of information from pharmacists or practitioners supplying drugs in areas where a particular drug problem arises. The legislation established an advisory council (the ACMD) to assist the Home Secretary in the preparation of controls and counter-measures; and aims to promote research and education in relation to the dangers of drug misuse (Stark et al., 1999).

Drugs which are controlled by this legislation are listed in schedule two of the Act and are divided into three classes, A, B and C (see Table 2.1). Crucially each drug is judged according to its 'relative harmfulness' and classified accordingly. However, the 1971 Act is not explicit in deciding how and why some drugs are more harmful than others. The Act uses the following criteria: firstly, whether the drug is being misused; secondly, whether it is likely to be misused; and, thirdly, whether its effects are likely to constitute a social problem. Although this raises problems in terms of explicitly determining which category a particular drug should go into, from the perspective of an enforcement agenda it is used to determine the criminal sanctions that are applied to the misuse of a particular drug (see Runciman, 1999) and seeks to deter people from drug use via criminal sanctions (House of Commons Science and Technology Committee 2005/2006).

Levine (2003) argues that all domestic drug policies are in fact examples of drug prohibition, which exist on a continuum between the most

TABLE 2.1   *Classification under the Misuse of Drugs Act (1971)*

Class A drugs

> Include: ecstasy, LSD, heroin, cocaine, crack, magic mushrooms (if prepared for use),
> amphetamines (if prepared for injection).
> Penalties for possession: up to seven years in prison, or an unlimited fine, or both.
> Penalties for dealing: up to life in prison, or an unlimited fine, or both.

Class B drugs

> Include: cannabis, amphetamines, Methylphenidate (Ritalin), Pholcodine.
> Penalties for possession: up to five years in prison, or an unlimited fine, or both.
> Penalties for dealing: up to 14 years in prison, or an unlimited fine, or both.

Class C drugs

> Include: tranquilisers, some painkillers, GHB (Gamma hydroxybutyrate), ketamine.
> Penalties for possession: up to two years in prison, or an unlimited fine, or both.
> Penalties for dealing: up to 14 years in prison, or an unlimited fine, or both.

Offences under the Act include:

- Possession of a controlled substance unlawfully.
- Possession of a controlled substance with intent to supply it.
- Supplying or offering to supply a controlled drug (even where no charge is made for the drug).
- Allowing premises you occupy or manage to be used unlawfully for the purpose of producing or supplying controlled drugs.

Drug trafficking (supply) attracts serious punishment including life imprisonment for Class A offences.

To enforce this law the police have special powers to stop, detain and search people on the 'reasonable suspicion' that they are in possession of a controlled drug.

Source: drugs.homeoffice.gov.uk/drugs-laws/misuse-of-drugs-act/

punitive (the USA) and the most liberal (the Netherlands) (see Table 2.2). All other western countries fall somewhere between these two. Levine argues that, despite the spread of drug prohibition around the world via the United Nations (and the dominant views of the USA in the process), the aim of global drug prohibition is facing a number of crises. Levine identifies the following as the crises in question: harm reduction within drug prohibition (see Chapter 4), the growing opposition to punitive drug policies, and the widespread use of cannabis around the world (see below).

In line with Levine's (2003) argument we can see that the British approach sits somewhere mid-point on the prohibition continuum between the USA and the Netherlands, but probably moving towards the 'liberal' end of the spectrum. This was initially demonstrated by the decision to reclassify cannabis to Class 'C' although the arguments about the appropriateness of this have continued with it now being reclassified to Class B. This demonstrates quite well the political uncertainty to be found in addressing some of these issues.

TABLE 2.2   *Prohibition as a continuum*

USA	United Kingdom	Netherlands
Criminalised drug prohibition	**British System**	**Decriminalised and regulated drug prohibition**
Prosecution of all drug use	Police emphasis on class 'A' drugs	Distinction between 'hard' and 'soft' drugs
Prohibit medical use of cannabis	Medical trials for use of THC	Prosecution of class 'A' drug dealers and suppliers
Long prison sentences for repeated possession, use and small scale possession	Increased use of cautioning/ non-prosecution for small amounts of cannabis for personal use	Prosecution of smugglers, dealers and commercial growers of large quantities of cannabis
	Since 1997 drug using criminals prioritised for drug treatment	Cafés licensed to sell small quantities of cannabis

The development of the 'British System' of drug control

It is useful to look at these issues and to discuss them within the context of what is called the 'British System', a 'term used to categorise the form of drug control policy established in Britain by the 1926 Rolleston Report. In general it is taken to mean a medically based system of prescribing opiates, often on a long term basis' (Berridge, 2005: 7). Despite the definition given by Berridge, the British System is not easy to describe or to encapsulate in short pithy sentences; 'one minute you can see it clearly; the next minute it seems to have vanished, and you realise you're not looking in the right place' (Strang and Gossop, 2005b: 1). Whilst substitute prescribing has been an important and constant feature of the system, what has changed is the professional contexts in which this is delivered, the attitudes of the practitioners involved, and the focus of government.

The 'British System' under New Labour

The key features of the British System and their legislative and policy connections in respect to aspects of care and control can be seen in the following examples (see Strang and Gossop, 2005a; 2005b):

Aspects of care

- the role of specialist drug clinics (Department of Health via the National Treatment Agency)
- the involvement of general practitioners/primary care (Shared Care Protocols)
- public health responses (needle exchange)
- community drug teams (NHS and Community Care Act 1990)

- substitute prescribing (Community Drugs Teams, GPs, pharmacies)
- harm minimisation approaches (voluntary and statutory sector providers)
- self-help (completely independent and self-funding)
- non-statutory sector involvement (for example charities) and contractual arrangements with DATs, CDPs, Supporting People Consortia.

Aspects of control

- a tougher focus on Class A drugs (the Home Office via the National Treatment Agency)
- new cross-regional police 'hit squads' to break up middle drug markets, the link in the chain between traffickers and local dealers
- new aftercare and throughcare services to improve community access to treatment and ensure that people leaving prison and treatment avoid the revolving door back into addiction and offending
- the move towards coercing people into treatment (Probation working in partnership with Community Drug Teams and other providers to test and provide services for drug using offenders).

The British approach has in the past been seen to be a model of tolerance, by on the one hand trying to deter people from using drugs and on the other trying to help them if they do. This harm minimisation approach rather than producing a 'system' has given rise to a patchwork of responses to a range of problems faced by drug users. Whilst the British System has always provided medically orientated services for substitute prescribing (see Chapter 4), other agencies have developed particularly in the non-statutory charitable sector to provide a range of support services for this group of people. Over time it had become recognised that dealing with these other issues is key to effective working with drug users, but there was little consistency nationally. The National Treatment Agency was set up by New Labour as a specialist Health Authority to work through DATs in the commissioning and developing of services to national standards via its Models of Care Framework (see Chapter 7). The aims of National Service Frameworks are to produce national consistency, coherence, local and national accountability, flexibility and the maximisation of resources (see Pycroft, 2005). Although working under the auspices of the Department of Health there are strong links with the Home Office, and in line with New Labour policy generally there is an emphasis on dealing with crime and anti-social behaviour. This has seen an increase in coercing people into treatment, as well as drug testing for all arrestees. This approach raises a number of ethical and practical issues. Firstly, given the biopsychosocial nature of addiction, and the reality of relapse, is there a place for criminal justice interventions in dealing with addiction? Secondly, there is the problem of what criminologists such as Garland (2001) argue is the case of more and more health and welfare agencies becoming incorporated into a criminal justice agenda (see Chapter 8 for a discussion on coerced interventions).

> What should the role of health and social welfare agencies be within the criminal justice system? Is it for example appropriate to be involved in punishing offenders through coerced interventions?

Reviewing relative harmfulness and differential prohibition

It can be seen that there is an interface between the law and order and helping agenda in respect of drug use, and that the emphases of this agenda between care and control vary over time. The dominance of a law and order agenda within New Labour policy means that a wide range of agencies is now involved in enforcing differential prohibition. As such we can define differential prohibition as a complex of laws, policies and procedures that involve the sanctioned control of the availability of some psychoactive substances for personal, medical and scientific reasons. The sanction and control arising from this prohibition are enforced through criminal law, civil law and governance. It is important that the concept of differential prohibition should be based upon the best evidence that can be provided to government and so ensure a democratic legitimacy for any legislative response (Stokes et al., 2001). Relative harmfulness is a useful and reasonable concept but one which needs to be developed and the Runciman Report (1999: 5) suggests that harm may be assessed on the basis of four factors: firstly, both the acute short term and chronic long term toxicity of the drug; secondly, risks due to the route of use; thirdly, the extent to which the drug controls behaviour in the form of addiction; and fourthly, the ease of stopping. This approach would allow for a more comprehensive analysis of individual drugs and the means by which they are consumed. What it does not do is explicitly take into account the risks to other people coming from drug use.

Pulling together the themes: cannabis and alcohol – a case study

These two drugs provide a useful comparison because they are both sedatives, have some differing effects, are both widely used, and are (or in the case of cannabis, becoming) socially acceptable. It is because of this increasing usage that the World Drug Report in 2006 (UNODC, 2006) paid particular attention to cannabis. The report estimated that 162 million people use cannabis annually, that it is produced in 176 countries, and that it raises concerns about the increased market share of some of the more potent forms of cannabis. Global production of cannabis fell in the 1980s and then rose again in the 1990s with increased demand. The report took the view that 'harmful characteristics of cannabis are no longer that different from those of other plant based drugs such as cocaine and heroin' (UNODC, 2006: 2). However, it is not possible to simply talk about 'cannabis' or 'alcohol' as there are variants of each with differing strengths and thus differing effects. In Tables 2.3 and 2.4, the differences become clear.

TABLE 2.3   *Types of cannabis*

- Resin – scraped and compressed from dry plants (accounts for 60% sales)
- Herbal – dried leaves (accounts for 40% sales)

  - Traditional leaf, flowering tops, leaves
  - Sinsemilla higher potency made from flowering tops of unfertilised female plants.

- Cannabis oil – solvent percolated through resin (accounts for less than 1% of usage)
- The main psychoactive component is delta-tetrahydrocannabinol (THC)
- Preparations vary greatly in potency with wide variations between plant varieties and content of THC.

TABLE 2.4   *Alcoholic beverages and their strengths*

Types of alcoholic beverage	Strength
Beers/Lagers	3–9%
Wine	8–14%
Fortified wine	Approx 20%
Spirits	40–80%
Homebrew	Variable

Cannabis use

The increased popularity and acceptability of this drug is demonstrated by the research which found that within the UK approximately 90% of men and women born between 1945 and 1949 report never having used cannabis whereas more than 50% born between 1980 and 1984 report cannabis use (Hickman et al., 2007). This is supported by the British Crime Survey (Home Office, 2000), which found that cannabis is the UK's most widely used illicit drug and is particularly prevalent amongst younger people. For 16 to 59 year olds the survey found that 27% had tried cannabis in their lifetime, with 9% in the last year and 6% in the last month, compared with 16 to 29 year olds of whom 44% had used it in their lifetime with 22% in the last year and 14% in the last month.

Within your peer group is cannabis a socially acceptable drug? Give some reasons for why it is acceptable or why it is not.

When making a comparison between the relative harmfulness of the two drugs (and allowing for variations in type) we can make the following observations of short and long term effects. Firstly, both lead to psychomotor impairment of balance and movement with an increased risk of accidents. Secondly, both cause lengthened reaction times which are dose related and so can cause problems such as road traffic accidents. Thirdly, this is linked to an impairment of judgement, and increased risk taking, and for alcohol increased aggressiveness. Fourthly, both drugs cause emotional changes and a decreased reaction to social expectations, with alcohol causing a significant risk of violence towards self and others. Alcohol is linked with a wide range of physical and mental health problems, whereas although treatment may be required for cannabis use, the health problems are similar to those for smoking tobacco (see Roffman and Stephens, 2006.)

Although it can be seen that there are many similarities between these two drugs, alcohol is particularly problematic because it is associated with such a wide range of medical, psychological and social issues and has the propensity to cause aggressive and violent behaviour. The Alcohol Harm Reduction Strategy for England (AHRSE) outlines some of the costs from alcohol use and includes 1.2 million violent incidents, 360,000 incidents of domestic violence, increased anti-social behaviour and fear of crime, expenditure of £95 million on alcohol treatment, over 30,000 hospital admissions for ADS, up to 22,000 premature deaths per annum, up to 1000 suicides, up to 17 million working days lost through alcohol related absence, up to 1.3 million children affected by parental alcohol problems and with marriages twice as likely to end in divorce (Cabinet Office, 2004).

The Licensing Act (2003)

If we take the notion of relative harmfulness and apply this to alcohol in terms of its toxicity, prevalence of misuse and harm to society, then clearly within the context of the Misuse of Drugs Act this is a dangerous drug; however, rather than seeking to control and disrupt supply, and curtail use, the Licensing Act (2003) effectively does the opposite by liberalising supply and availability. This has given rise to the potential for pubs and bars be to open 24 hours a day.

Under the legislation it is incumbent upon Local Authorities to make decisions about licensing hours which are best suited to their locality and in so doing they must take into account the imperative to prevent crime and disorder, and public nuisance, and to protect the public and children from harm. The government was primarily concerned to deal with the crime and disorder that arose in towns and cities at 'drinking up' time, when groups of people would rush their drinks before the pubs and bars shut and would all turn out onto the streets at the same time. It was argued that staggered leaving times and the abandonment of 'last orders' would help the work of the police in ensuring public safety. There is evidence to suggest that in fact this has not worked entirely in the way it was intended. Roberts and Eldridge (2007), in research for the Institute of Alcohol Studies, found a huge variation in opinion across the UK as to whether the staggering of closing hours was having a beneficial effect.

However, irrespective of the specific public safety aspects the work of Edwards et al. (1994) and Babor et al. (2003) clearly demonstrates that there is a correlation between the total amount of alcohol consumed within a population and the level of a wide range of alcohol related problems in that population. The supply and availability of a drug, in this case alcohol, is controlled through licensing schemes, age restrictions and pricing controls. Pricing has been an extremely effective way of reducing smoking within the population (see Edwards et al., 1994 and Babor et al., 2003).

> Are you prepared to pay more for your alcohol in the interests of public health? What do you see as the arguments for and against this proposition?

We can see that as cannabis use has become more widespread then concerns about its effects have become more prevalent, for example, in relation to mental health problems and addiction. However, as compared with alcohol 'the acute toxicity of cannibinoids are very low: they are very safe drugs and no deaths have been directly attributed to their recreational or therapeutic use' (British Medical Association evidence in Runciman, 1999) whereas 'social customs and economic interests should not blind us to the fact that alcohol is a toxic substance ... no other commodity sold for ingestion, not even tobacco, has such wide ranging adverse physical effects' (Babor et al., 2003: 4).

Links with mental health problems

One of the main reasons for reclassifying cannabis back to Class B under the Misuse of Drugs Act (1971) was the perceived link with mental health problems, particularly in relation to the use of the more potent Sinsemilla (also known as Skunk). There is a clear relationship between alcohol and mental health problems (Meltzer, 1995), with between 22% and 44% of adult psychiatric inpatients experiencing problems with alcohol and drugs and the most severely dependent drinkers reporting the greatest number of mental and physical health problems (Gossop et al., 2003). Gossop (2000) argues that there is no convincing evidence that cannabis causes mental health problems and that, given that the prevalence of psychosis in the general population is about 1%, it is obvious that some cannabis users will develop psychosis. He also makes the point that cannabis use may exacerbate existing problems; however, it is also the case that cannabis may form a part of poly drug use which may exacerbate the risks of developing mental health problems.

The Gateway Theory

The Gateway Theory has been one of the major arguments against the legalisation or decriminalisation of cannabis. The hypothesis is that cannabis use leads to the use of harder drugs. This theory is based upon the observation that hard drug users have a history of cannabis use. This theory was reviewed by Runciman (1999) who argued that this is partly linked to the drug markets in which dealers encourage people to try other drugs and that the earlier the initiation into cannabis then the more likely people are to progress to other drugs. However, any sustainable theory has to show the strong probability of progression and not just that a heroin user has also used cannabis. It is evident from the statistics the vast majority of cannabis users do not progress, otherwise there would be far greater numbers of 'hard' drug users than there actually are.

One of the key challenges for state and society is to determine what is an acceptable level of use and availability of particular psychoactive substances. In addition, can we be serious about reducing tobacco usage, through banning smoking in public places, but at the same time liberalise the use of cannabis? These are difficult questions that go to the heart of citizenship and freedoms within society but are nonetheless important to address. Both student and practitioner need to ask smart questions; for example, when talking about cannabis or alcohol what are we talking about, given the differing strengths and types of each, and different patterns of use? Government has a duty to protect people from harm, and drugs cause an inordinate amount of human suffering, and so at the very least a reasonable and rationale approach to classifying harm is required.

Useful resources

In addition to those outlined above there are a number of key pieces of legislation that relate not only to the enforcement of prohibitive measures in respect of drug use, but also to the rehabilitation of people experiencing drug problems, for example:

Dual Diagnosis Protocols (see Chapter 5)
Mental Health Act (2007)
NHS and Community Care Act (1990)
Supporting People (supported housing)
Go to www.alcoholconcern.org.uk to read about the plans by the Scottish Parliament to introduce minimum pricing for alcohol

3

From Disease to Dependency Syndrome

The aims of this chapter are to:

- outline the disease conceptions of addiction, their strengths and weaknesses
- discuss the development of dependence syndromes, their strengths and weaknesses
- examine how the notion of dependence syndromes has informed the classification of drug and alcohol problems.

The problem of language and semantics has had huge effects on the substance misuse field, none more so than the concept of addiction as an illness or disease. The idea of disease and its implications for those who suffer from it, and the role of society in preventing and treating it, become bound up within a nexus of competing cultural mores and norms, scientific evidence and political decision making. Throughout most of the twentieth century there was a lack of conceptual clarity in understanding and defining alcohol dependence and its related problems (Thom, 1999; Li et al., 2007a) and mainly because the accepted disease conception was the one promulgated by Alcoholics Anonymous (see below) which developed out of a self-help approach rather than scientific endeavour.

In what ways might addiction be viewed as a disease?

The disease of alcoholism

According to Lindstrom (1992: 50) the notion of alcohol dependency as the disease of 'alcoholism' originated in the eighteenth century, and was very much developed and promoted by the Temperance Movement in the nineteenth and early twentieth centuries but really gained ground after the Second World War, particularly through the work of the World Health Organisation. This approach has been promulgated by Alcoholics Anonymous (AA) (and more latterly by Narcotics Anonymous (NA) and other twelve step programmes) who have had considerable influence in defining the idea and by forging a partnership with the medical profession (Thom, 1999).

It is difficult to underestimate just how significant disease conceptions of addiction have been upon policy and practice, particularly in respect of 'alcoholism'. The particular historical events that gave rise to the Temperance Movements by a coalition of evangelical Christians and public health reformers are well documented (see Heather and Robertson, 1981; 1997). In particular, in an age that saw a move towards public health interventions and an ongoing recognition of the destructive power of alcohol, general practitioners, working in the most deprived urban areas, endorsed a disease perspective. Thom (1999) notes that it was the propagandist value of the disease approach which was more important than any appeal to scientific validity and as such the concept was left deliberately vague.

In essence the disease concept, which at times has been highly symbolic in nature, has acted as a rallying cry and as an organising construct for action in the alcohol field (Thom, 1999). Given the origins of the concept within a radicalised, well organised and evangelical Christianity it should come as no surprise that the concept would appear philosophically, organisationally and purposively Christian in nature, although the Twelve Step movement has distanced itself in its public pronouncements (see the AA website) from a purely Christian perspective, seeking to include a generic faith perspective and an approach to include those who have none.

Alcoholics Anonymous

The disease perspective, as developed throughout the twentieth century, is most clearly linked with the organisation and mission of AA and NA. The bases of AA/NA are the Twelve Traditions and the Twelve Steps (see Table 3.1) which encapsulate the essentially Christian, communal, non-hierarchical, self-help and missionary orientation of the movement. The Twelve Traditions outline the ways in which AA/NA are organised: it is a mission statement that states the need for group support under the ultimate authority of a loving God, with leaders who are trusted servants but do not govern. Personal recovery from alcoholism is dependent upon unity within the group, with the only requirement for membership of the group being a desire to stop drinking/using drugs. The Traditions emphasise that the primary purpose of each group is to carry its message to the alcoholic/ addict who still suffers. Autonomy is seen as crucial to the mission of the groups so that they cannot be compromised in anyway by endorsements, money and property, and diverted from their primary purpose. Although there are many rehabilitation programmes based upon the principle of AA/NA, the organisation itself will not enter into contractual arrangements to provide services as this would potentially change the nature of the help that is being offered; neither will they comment upon any issues in the public domain with the need to main anonymity as the spiritual basis for the work that they do.

TABLE 3.1   *The Twelve Steps of Alcoholics Anonymous*

1	We admitted we were powerless over alcohol – that our lives had become unmanageable.
2	Came to believe that a Power greater than ourselves could restore us to sanity.
3	Made a decision to turn our will and our lives over to the care of God as we understood Him.
4	Made a searching and fearless moral inventory of ourselves.
5	Admitted to God, to ourselves, and to another human being the exact nature of our wrongs.
6	Were entirely ready to have God remove all these defects of character.
7	Humbly asked Him to remove our shortcomings.
8	Made a list of all persons we had harmed, and became willing to make amends to them all.
9	Made direct amends to such people wherever possible, except when to do so would injure them or others.
10	Continued to take personal inventory and when we were wrong promptly admitted it.
11	Sought through prayer and meditation to improve our conscious contact with God, as we understood Him, praying only for knowledge of His will for us and the power to carry that out.
12	Having had a spiritual awakening as the result of these Steps, we tried to carry this message to alcoholics, and to practise these principles in all our affairs.

There is no formal 'AA definition' of alcoholism, but AA information (www.alcoholics-anonymous.org.uk) describes it as a *physical compulsion, coupled with a mental obsession,* meaning that alcoholics have a distinct physical desire to consume alcohol beyond their capacity to control it, and contrary to common sense: 'We not only had an abnormal craving for alcohol but we frequently yielded to it at the worst possible times. We did not know when (or how) to stop drinking. Often we did not seem to have sense enough to know when not to begin'.

Alcoholics Anonymous and biopsychosociality

What this disease conceptualisation of addiction provides us with is a prototype biopsychosocial paradigm fused with a religious perspective. Within this model the biological components clearly refer to physical compulsion, the psychological components to obsession, and the social aspects to recovery from the problem. Inherent within this model is the idea of the addict as being different from the non-addict. The emphasis is on a new moral awakening to overcome the problem, which is markedly different to the Moral Model which had seen addicts as people who used alcohol because they chose to drink in a problematic fashion. This capacity for rational people to choose makes them worthy of moral condemnation (see Lindstrom, 1992) and is a theme that is still obvious within contemporaneous criminal justice responses to drug addiction (see Chapters 7 and 8). However, the clear message arising from this new approach was that alcoholics are ill, they are suffering from a disease, and they need help not condemnation.

> To what extent do you think that drug use is a rational choice, and do people choose to become addicted to particular substances?

Picking up on the issue of the disease model lacking clarity, Heather and Robertson (1997) argue that within this approach it is possible to identify three main types of disease theories: firstly, alcoholism as a pre-existent physical abnormality; secondly, alcoholism as an a mental illness or psychopathology; and, thirdly, alcoholism as an acquired addiction or dependence. Although there is no clear demarcation between these approaches we can infer that there are key issues here of genetic influences and psychiatric disturbance as well as developmental attributes. Whilst Heather and Robertson (1981, 1997) seek to dismiss disease approaches from a psychological perspective, it is important to realise that those approaches have made a significant contribution to the process of learning about and understanding the nature of alcohol and drug problems.

Despite the lack of conceptual clarity Lindstrom (1992) cites Sobell and Sobell (1977) who argue that the classical disease model can be summarised using the following assumptions:

- that there is a unitary phenomenon that can be identified as alcoholism; alcoholics and pre-alcoholics are essentially different from non-alcoholics
- that alcoholics may sometimes experience an irresistible physical craving for alcohol

- that alcoholics gradually develop a process called 'loss of control' over drinking and possibly an inability to stop drinking
- that alcoholism is a permanent and irreversible progressive disease which follows an inexorable development through a distinct series of phases.

Disease and personal responsibility

The controversy about the nature of addiction, and whether it is a disease process, or what the components or course of that disease might be has serious consequences for individuals and society. At the heart of these issues are ideas of personal responsibility and the degree to which individuals can be culpable for their actions. If I am addicted to alcohol or heroin, is this a rational choice that I have made and given the potential harm to myself, my family and my community should I be punished for this behaviour, and other people be deterred from doing the same thing? Or is it an illness or disease that requires treatment, compassion and understanding from my family, community and the state? This issue of personal responsibility lies at the heart of many of the debates: consider the discussions over whether heavy drinkers should be given a liver transplant or whether smokers should have access to health services if they continue to smoke.

Disease and the 'sick role'

The idea that addicts needed help rather than condemnation was promulgated by a number of organisations who incorporated an element of biological based thinking into their roles and missions. The Temperance Movement, the medical profession, the WHO, and Alcoholics Anonymous have all had a significant influence on developing services for people with alcohol (and latterly illicit drug) problems. A consequence of this disease perspective has been to exempt the individual suffering from this disease from personal responsibility. How can they be responsible when they are suffering from a disease? This approach would appear to be double edged insofar as its humanitarian basis has clearly influenced the provision of services for people who are suffering, but has abdicated them from responsibility for that suffering. In sociological terms this has been encapsulated in Talcott Parsons' sick role (Bilton et al., 2002), whereby the individual is exempted from normal social roles and responsibilities by virtue of his or her illness. This, however, is relative to the nature and severity of the illness, so the more severe the illness the greater the exemption. This exemption has to be legitimated by a doctor as the authority on what actually constitutes sickness and which serves the social function of protecting society against malingerers who attempt to remain in the sick role longer than social expectations allow. This usually happens so that the sick person can acquire the secondary gains, or additional privileges, afforded to ill persons. The sick person is not held responsible for his or her condition because the illness is usually thought to be beyond his or her own control.

In return for these exemptions, the individual suffering from illness has certain obligations. Firstly, the individual should try to get well and recognize that being sick is undesirable and that exemption is only temporary and conditional. Secondly, the sick person has to seek help from a technically competent physician to assist them in the process of getting well and to cooperate with the physician in the process of trying to get well.

The Twelve Step model seems to take this issue of responsibility to an extreme, by declaring that addicts are 'powerless' over their behaviour, that there is something fundamental and pathological in their makeup that prevents them from drinking like 'non-alcoholics'. This approach of gaining control by giving up control is known as the control paradox (Baugh, 1988). Humphreys (2004: 39) argues that this issue of 'powerlessness' and the need to surrender to a 'higher power' is misunderstood insofar that it is simply an acknowledgement of the limits of human control 'rather than an endorsement of irresponsibility'. People joining AA/NA are encouraged only to try and take control of that which they are able to do, and in that respect the Twelve Steps represent a series of behavioural stages that allow an individual to slowly assume more responsibility for their own actions. In this respect the AA/NA group is very similar to other therapeutic groups (see Yalom, 2005) insofar as the frightened, anxious and concerned individual starts by being entirely dependent upon the group as their external locus of control, which then becomes more internal with recovery. As people recover they are then able to start thinking about helping others, but the group is essential to ongoing well-being and the avoidance of relapse.

In addition, although politically and legislatively alcohol has been dealt with very differently from other psychoactive substances (see Chapter 2), at the clinical and treatment level the development of understanding alcohol problems has also led the way to developing a theory and practice for all drugs. Given the widespread nature of alcohol use over the course of history, as compared with other drugs such as opiates, the development of understanding alcohol use, notions of misuse, addiction, the problems therein and recovery from those problems provides useful insights into other drugs as well.

There is a sense in which the disease model as propounded by AA is a model based upon clinical observation, particularly in relation to notions of craving, a loss of control and the rapid reinstatement of symptoms following relapse.

These medico-psychological constructs have continued through into the dependence syndrome. But also, given the status of Twelve Step programmes within the treatment field, there has been an ongoing interest in the field of spirituality and religion both as a protective factor against, and as a solution to, addiction (see Cook, 2004; Humphreys and Gifford, 2006).

The strengths and weaknesses of the disease perspective

As a prototype biopsychosocial model the disease perspective cannot be easily dismissed as it has paved the way for the development of helping services, many of which operate on a self-help basis, entirely free at the point of delivery and entirely accessible when people need them the most. Many 'professional' organisations have a great deal to learn from them. The biopsychosocial elements of this model may not be fully developed but they have stimulated a research agenda into the complex nature of addiction, which has gradually identified some of the core components of the problem.

The disease model does, however, have some weaknesses which will be discussed here and in the next chapter on psychology. From a clinical or practitioner perspective it is evident from the Twelve Steps and the traditions of AA that an important part of the process of recovery from the disease of alcoholism is to actually admit and acknowledge that you have that disease. Step One is to acknowledge powerlessness over behaviour, and in Step Two to recognise what psychologists would call an external locus of control, and what AA calls a 'higher power'. Not recognising or acknowledging that you are an 'alcoholic' is seen to be a denial of the problem, and 'being in denial' is a phrase that has passed into popular parlance.

This approach can have a double-edged effect: I have worked with people who were very often confused, anxious, guilty and angry about their behaviour around alcohol or drugs, and could understand why they continued to engage in this problematic behaviour even when it had such severe consequences. What the disease label can often give people at their lowest ebb is reassurance; I have heard people express their relief at discovering that they have a 'disease' and that other people have it too and that they are not alone. The label and the thinking that goes with it allow them to then make sense of what is happening to them. When people are highly anxious they want certainty and they get this through AA. However, the danger here is that this can become a self-fulfilling prophecy and that people can start to become the stereotype of that which they have become labelled with. We will look at this in more detail in the next chapter, but this labelling for example can lead to a kind of circular thinking, whereby an individual expresses a concern about their drinking behaviour and you engage in a discussion about why they drink in the way that they do, to which the answer comes back 'because I'm an alcoholic'. It would seem that the disease perspective can become a generalisation that militates against people looking for subtle antecedent cues, or understanding the learned basis of behaviour, all of which falls within the domain of psychological models.

In addition to labelling, this perspective encourages a 'one size fits all' approach, with an emphasis on recognising and diagnosing who are the real 'alcoholics' and thus with another emphasis on complete abstinence as the only realistic outcome from treatment. This raises a number of important issues not just for clinical practice but also for policy makers and the commissioners of services as well. The implications of this approach are that there is an emphasis on heavy end 'alcoholics' and not a prevention agenda, and also of course it abdicates the alcohol industry and government from any blame concerning the supply and availability of alcohol. It is no wonder that the alcohol industry has been keen to endorse the disease perspective (Thom, 1999).

Within this approach there was then little understanding of problematic drinking or other drug use as being dimensional in nature. There was an understanding that the problems that alcoholics/addicts experience are directly related to the disease process, and that once the drug use stops all areas of their lives recover (McKay and McClellan, 1998). This of course necessitates a negative view of relapse because according to this logic even one drink or drug use will usher in the symptoms of the disease (see the section on the Abstinence Violation Effect (AVE) in the next chapter), but once again this is an aspect of labelling whereby the individual says that 'I might just as well be hung for a sheep as for a lamb' and thus carries on drinking because that is how alcoholics behave.

> Have you tried dieting, or giving up smoking or drinking, and then eaten more than you intended or had a cigarette or a drink? How did this affect your motivation and intentions to cut down or quit?

Of great significance in the history of the disease concept were findings by Sobell and Sobell and the Rand Report (1974) (both cited by Heather and Robertson, 1997) of controlled and unproblematic levels of drinking by individuals who had been diagnosed as alcoholic and had been through treatment. This evidence and the emergence of psychology from the shadow of psychoanalysis (Yalom, 1980) particularly in relation to cognitive processes started to challenge the unitary one size fits all approach.

The Alcohol Dependence Syndrome

In 1976 Griffith Edwards and Milton Gross (Edwards and Gross, 1976) provisionally outlined and argued for a new conceptual understanding of alcohol dependence based upon the idea of dependence as a syndrome. This was a revolutionary approach which marked a distinct shift away from a disease perspective which had been in the ascendancy during most of the previous twentieth century. It also paved the way for a new plethora of approaches to the prevention and treatment of alcohol and drug related problems. This new approach sought to clarify the clinical dimension of problems arising from alcohol use and to generate research that would inform new and accurate diagnostic criteria and improved treatments (Li et al., 2007a). The principles underlying the Alcohol Dependence Syndrome (ADS) were rapidly adopted by the World Health Organisation (WHO), and formed the basis of the classification of both alcohol and drug problems in the *International Classification of Diseases* (ICD-10) and the *Diagnostic and Statistical Manual* (DSM-IV) of the American Psychiatric Association. Both of these classification systems contain elements of the original ADS, although arguments remain about the specific criteria used to identify the syndrome and its progression (Li et al., 2007a).

Interestingly both the ADS and the disease approach have arisen out of clinical practice, and the need to help people with alcohol problems. Edwards and Gross (1976: 1058) stated that their provisional description of the syndrome was based upon 'clinical impression', in the same way that the disease approach is the collective wisdom of fellow 'alcoholics' and addicts trying to understand and respond to what they understand is happening to them through their drug use. The crucial difference here is the role of professional and lay science, and interestingly Orford (2008), in arguing for a new research paradigm in the addictions, cites the need to listen to addicts' understandings of the problems that they are experiencing (see Chapter 8).

It was the development of the ADS which really opened up a whole new vista of research opportunities and thinking around the issues related initially to alcohol, but then to drug use generally. It has been critiqued by psychologists such as Heather and Robertson (1981; 1997) as being no more than a continuation of disease theories that they argue represents 'the most important recent event in the history of disease conceptions of alcoholism (Heather and Robertson, 1981: 15). Edwards and Gross (1976: 1058) argued that in forming a clinical impression about people presenting with alcohol problems 'no assumptions need to be made about the cause or the pathological process' that is at work.

The classification of problems serves a number of philosophical, methodological and practical functions which have been well expressed by Babor (1992). He argues that the usefulness of diagnostic criteria and systems of classification stems from their ability to make clinical decisions, estimating the prevalence, understanding the aetiology of the problem, and facilitating scientific communication. Above all, this then provides a common frame of reference that researchers and practitioners can work with. However, as Li et al. (2007a) point out, because of the historical nature of the evolution of approaches to understanding alcohol problems and what is meant by terminology such as 'disease', a greater clarity is still lacking.

Edwards and Gross described seven provisional criteria that constituted the ADS. They 'take the term syndrome to mean no more than the concurrence of phenomena. Not all the elements need always be present, nor always present with the same intensity' (1976: 1058).

1 Narrowing of the drinking repertoire For most people who do not have an alcohol problem, their consumption of alcohol will vary over time and be dependent upon mood and leisure and social activities. Drinking is cued by a number of internal and external factors. As a person starts to drink more heavily then she or he may drink on more occasions. As dependence develops the cues associated with drinking may become more related to the avoidance of alcohol withdrawal and thus the personal drinking repertoire may become increasingly narrowed. Irrespective of the social context the individual begins to drink the same amount across all situations. Edwards and Gross refer to the drinking behaviour becoming stereotyped, whereby it fits with a pattern to maintain high blood/alcohol concentrations; for example early morning drinking to avoid 'the shakes'. However, they also argue that despite this stereotyping effect there is always the capacity for some variation with the syndrome being 'pictured as subtle and plastic rather than as something set hard' (1976: 1059).

2 Salience of drink seeking behaviour With this process of stereotyping, the individual is giving greater priority to maintaining their alcohol intake, to the point whereby the drinking continues despite the negative consequences of ill health and social difficulties and indeed conflict within the individual themselves over this behaviour.

3   Increased tolerance to alcohol   The central nervous system develops tolerance to alcohol, which is demonstrated by individuals being able to operate at blood alcohol concentrations that are far higher than for someone who has not developed tolerance.

4   Repeated withdrawal symptoms   Withdrawal symptoms occur when blood alcohol concentrations drop, and include a range of symptoms from nausea, vomiting, tremor and headaches through to muscle cramps, sleep disturbance, serious convulsions (that can lead to death) and hallucinations.

5   Relief or avoidance of withdrawal symptoms by further drinking   As mentioned above the drinker may realise that by utilising 'the hair of the dog' that they can keep their blood alcohol concentrations at a level to avoid experiencing withdrawal symptoms.

6   Subjective awareness of compulsion to drink   This compulsion to drink is often described as 'craving' and 'loss of control' both of which are key concepts in the disease model. Edwards and Gross argue that control may be impaired rather than lost, and that some people may choose to give up control. This important area has been the subject of much research by psychologists who have looked at self-efficacy (situational confidence) as a key process in relapse prevention and management (see Chapter 5).

7   Reinstatement after abstinence   Edwards and Gross (1976: 1060) say that the rapid reinstatement of severe withdrawal symptoms and continued drinking after abstinence is 'one of the most puzzling features of addiction'.

The dimensional nature of addiction

Whilst Edwards and Gross (1976) clearly saw that alcohol dependence was biologically driven, they saw the need to separate out the sphere of problems, and this gave rise to the bi-axial basis of the ADS. Both DSM-IV and ICD utilise a bi-axial concept of addiction (see Table 8) which encapsulates a broad range of Alcohol Use Disorders in two categories: firstly, alcohol dependence is concerned with the pharmacological aspects of dependence (tolerance and withdrawal), maladaptive responses to alcohol (loss of control and compulsion to drink), and secondly, the severity of addiction (negative consequences, time spent obtaining alcohol or drinking).

In Figure 3.1, Drummond (1992) demonstrates this concept, and the ways in which the core constructs relate to each other. He postulates that those people in the lower left quadrant are those people in a population

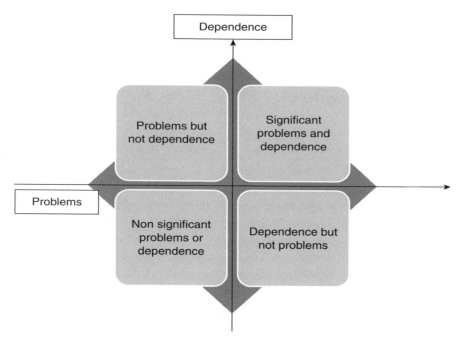

FIGURE 3.1   *The Dimensional Nature of the Alcohol Dependence Syndrome*
Source: Lader et al. (1992). By permission of Oxford University Press.

who use a substance, but do not experience significant problems or dependence with that use. Conversely those in the upper right quadrant are a typical 'clinical' population who experience high levels of both dependence and problems associated with their drug use. Those in the top left quadrant are people who experience problems but not necessarily a dependence associated with their substance use, for example those who drink and drive, or young people who drink heavily on a night out and end up in a fight. Finally, the bottom right quadrant represents people who are highly dependent but not experiencing significant problems. People on substitute prescriptions may fit into this category (see Chapter 4), and it is one of the key aims of the harm reduction agenda. Drummond argues (and in keeping with the premise of the ADS) that these quadrants do not represent distinct all or nothing categories, as problems and dependence exist on a continuum of severity.

Drummond (1992) argues that the importance of the ADS lies in the fact that it has provided a common frame of reference for clinicians and researchers to work to; it has moved us away from the unitary view of addiction provided by classical disease models, and perhaps most importantly of all, has opened up a whole new research agenda. This has been possible because people with alcohol problems are a heterogeneous group, who experience varying levels of severity in their problems. A 'one size fits all' approach is neither scientifically nor ethically valid in working with individuals who experience these problems.

Li et al. (2007b: 1537) argue that over the last 30 years 'the conceptual validity of the alcohol dependence syndrome has been demonstrated' but challenge the bi-axial nature of problems and dependence. They point to evidence that suggests that rather than having two distinct dimensions, namely dependence and problems, that alcohol disorders exist along a single continuum of severity. Problems are thus dose related insofar as developing an Alcohol Use Disorder increases significantly with the consumption of more than the recommended weekly limits for alcohol. This risk of dependence increases in a linear fashion with increased drinking, with both the volume and pattern of drinking contributing to it. However, this process is not clear as heavy drinking may lead to dependence, or dependence to heavy drinking, or both may operate in tandem (Babor et al., 2003).

Conclusion

Disease concepts of 'alcoholism' have had a crucial part to play in the development of practice, services and policy in response to problems associated with alcohol use. Initially those responses were based around an essentially Protestant Christian approach predicated upon a social gospel that saw the necessity of helping people to help themselves. The development of AA in 1935 has been of worldwide importance, through its own ways of working but also because of the influence that it has had on the development of other Twelve Step programmes as well. NA was founded in 1953 and Gamblers Anonymous in 1957. AA now has approximately 2.1 million members in 100,766 registered groups in 134 countries and NA has 20,000 registered groups in more than 100 countries. The presence and dedication of these organisations has clearly informed everyday 'commonsense' notions of what it means to be an 'alcoholic' or an 'addict'. In the same way that Hall (2006: 1530) argues that there is a 'popular understanding in the community of what it means to say that a disease or a disorder has a genetic basis', a 'folk genetics perspective', so too for addiction. Someone might be termed a 'real alcoholic', or in treatment centres you might hear the converse that someone is not a 'real alcoholic': this is the black and white categorisation that has been a product of the disease perspective.

The development of the ADS presented a watershed in the clinical approach to working with alcohol related issues, with the opportunity to do preventative work as well as deal with 'heavy end' drinkers. Again the development of this approach was essentially practical in nature, and paved the way for working more effectively with other substances as well. As research has continued then the ADS itself, 30 years down the line, is being reviewed particularly with reference to its bi-axial basis. In Chapter 6 we will be revisiting notions of disease in the light of findings from neurobiology and the unlocking of the human genome; however, both the disease perspective and the ADS were important in not dismissing some of the biological components of addiction, which have now assumed a new significance. While the ADS may continue to describe the symptoms experienced by excessive use of a substance it still does not tell us why, although we can appreciate in a more detailed way the importance of subjective awareness and social context. Developments in behaviourist and cognitive psychology then began to contribute to a mature understanding of how and why people change their problematic behaviour.

However, despite debates about the nature of addiction, and the place of personal responsibility, within the classical disease model which has seemingly been left behind in a mountain of scientific research there are a number of apparent paradoxes. We have already discussed gaining control by giving up control, but this also needs to be seen in the context of Twelve Step interventions having outcomes that are no better or worse than any other types of intervention (see Chapter 8). Both AA/NA and the ADS have developed based upon clinical observations, one set professional and one set not, but nonetheless many of those observations have a concurrence which has seen an historical and pragmatic alliance. These issues will be discussed further in Chapter 8, but for the above reasons AA/NA and their ilk cannot be easily dismissed.

Useful resources

Alcoholics Anonymous – www.alcoholics-anonymous.org.uk/
Diagnostic and Statistical Manual – IV – allpsych.com/disorders/dsm.html
International Classification of Diseases – 10 – www.who.int/classifications/icd/en/
Narcotics Anonymous – www.ukna.org/

4

Harm Reduction Approaches

The aims of this chapter are to:

- explain the concept of 'harm reduction' and the context in which it has arisen
- outline the main approaches to harm reduction including needle exchange and substitute prescribing
- discuss some of the tensions inherent within this approach.

A 'harm reduction' agenda sits within a public health approach, which seeks to develop policy and practice based upon 'scientific' evidence to both prevent problems and, where problems do arise, to intervene in the most effective way. In practice policies exist aimed at, firstly, universal prevention (Robson and Marlatt, 2006), which are the basis of the UN conventions, and the domestic legislation of the signatories to those conventions (in the UK the Misuse of Drugs Act (1971)) and, secondly, drug education in schools and public awareness campaigns. However, an epidemiological approach also indicates that within a general population some sub-populations may have an increased risk of developing or experiencing problems with drugs such as those with mental health problems, or those living in poverty, or homeless people (see Chapter 1). Therefore, selective interventions are required which are aimed at high risk groups, and the major impetus for the expansion of the harm reduction agenda in the UK was the identification of the link between injecting drug use and HIV infection in the 1980s.

The shift in clinical thinking from disease to dependence syndrome, and the identification of dependence/addiction as dimensional in nature, opened up the possibilities for a more comprehensive approach to dealing with the issues concerned. Rather than focusing on the 'heavy end' alcoholics or addicts the importance of preventative work was recognised, with an emphasis on the language of 'risk' (Berridge, 2002). Berridge identifies 'risk' as one of the core constructs within a chronic disease epidemiology based upon probabilistic statistics that have defined evidence based medicine and clinical effectiveness in the post-war years. There is clearly the risk of individuals developing a problem with illicit or legal drugs and there are further and enhanced risks involved of developing further and more complicated harms for individuals and communities.

Many of these health and social issues often involve fear, stigma and misunderstanding, and it is argued that, to address premature morbidity from preventable causes, scientific evidence based knowledge alone is not sufficient (Fry et al., 2008) and that a more value based approach is required. There are very real practical considerations involved in containing the spread of disease and other preventable harms, but these issues go to the heart of debates about individual rights, democracy, community and the power of the state to intervene in individual and community life.

In the same ways that the disease model of alcoholism focused on complete abstinence from alcohol use so drug treatment too had prioritised the elimination of drug use rather than preventing the adverse consequences of that use. Duke (2003) notes that during the 1980s a successful community public health agenda was operating which embraced the concepts of 'risk reduction' and 'harm minimisation', and 'harm reduction'. This was a pragmatic approach which incorporated the paradoxical themes of enforcement and punishment and harm minimisation and public health approaches and fitted well with the 'British System'. Consequently there has been a rapid development of harm reduction interventions to address the negative consequences of illicit and licit drug use for individuals and their communities, which has become an unnecessarily controversial issue as 'drug use control, or both harm reduction strategies are essential components of any modern treatment programme', (UNODC, 2008a: 1). Ball (2007) argues that the concepts, which tend to be used interchangeably, of 'harm reduction', 'risk reduction', 'harm minimisation', and 'vulnerability reduction', generate extremes of emotion, unlike virtually any other terms in the field of drug policy. He states that these responses (whether it is from people who see the efforts to control drugs being undermined, or drug legalisers who see opportunities for law reform, or practitioners who want to improve interventions) are not helped by the lack of a clear definition of what is meant by the term 'harm reduction'. We have already seen that Levine (2003) has argued that this harm reduction agenda, along with growing opposition to punitive approaches to dealing with drug users, is undermining the prohibitionist stance of the UN conventions and its signatories. According to Ball (2007: 684) 'the term has been used variously to describe a principle, concept, ideology, policy, strategy, set of interventions, target and movement'.

> In your opinion does a harm reduction agenda fit with the prohibitionist aims of the Misuse of Drugs Act (1971)?

These issues, and some of the tensions therein, are perhaps best highlighted by the publication of the Scottish Government's new drug policy, entitled *The Road to Recovery: A New Approach to Tackling Scotland's Drug Problem* (Scottish Government, 2008). They argue that this is 'a new approach to tackling problem drug use based firmly on the concept of recovery' which is 'a process through which an individual is enabled to move-on from their problem drug use towards a drug free life and become an active and contributing member of society' (2008: vi). Implicit within this approach is that, although substitute prescribing particularly for opiate users has been important in tackling drug use, and wider issues of HIV and hepatitis infection, there would seem to be a lack of services for people who want to choose to be completely drug free.

The controversy about harm reduction centres upon the fact that 'harm reduction can be viewed as the prevention of adverse consequences of illicit drug use without necessarily reducing their consumption' (Costigan et al., 2003: 35 cited in UNODC, 2008a: 1). The primary concerns of harm reduction are minimising the risks of contracting infectious diseases, the risk of overdose, or other negative consequences of substance use. Different strategies can focus on health issues or social, environmental and familial issues. However, despite being 25 years into the HIV epidemic, there is still no universally accepted definition – how 'harm' is defined is contentious – and all within debates about the necessity of a 'broad' versus 'narrow' approach. The latter is concerned with whether any approach can be included, including an attempt to reduce drug use, or whether it should be exclusively used in the reduction of harm (Ball, 2007).

In defining harm reduction, and within the context of the pragmatism of the 'British System', Robson and Marlatt (2006) take a broad view and argue that it covers a range of possible interventions with the common feature of these not being aimed at abstinence. This therefore includes using policy to encourage moderation or deter use, as well as working with individual drug/alcohol users to help manage their problems with more insight and the modification of public drug using or drinking environments. Whilst the focus of harm reduction approaches has been very much on the risks associated with illicit drugs, it is also increasingly being used as an approach in the alcohol field as well (Robson and Marlatt, 2006). In many ways the traditional approach to both prevention and harm reduction has been via public education through advertising campaigns and education in schools. The main themes associated with these approaches are summarised by Giesbrecht (2007), with the assumption that simply telling people about a risk or danger, or training them to be more aware, is an effective way of initiating behavioural change. These approaches are widely used and are largely non-controversial as they do not require structural change, or a reduced tax income for governments or profits for producers from licit drugs. As a consequence this approach is popular within the drinks industry but to date has not been shown to be effective in postponing, reducing consumption, or reducing high risk use or reducing rates of damage from alcohol.

This chapter will focus primarily upon harm reduction approaches with illicit drug use, although as will become evident, licit drugs such as alcohol have a major part to play in complex networks of causation.

Blood-borne viruses and needle exchange

Whilst a public health/harm reduction approach is used in the broad sense, it is more usually associated in the narrow sense with two approaches to working with injecting drug users, namely needle exchange and substitute prescribing to prevent the spread of disease via contaminated blood as well as the prevention of overdose and death (www.nta.nhs.uk/about_treatment/ Types_of_treatment.aspx). According to Solberg et al. (2002), drug injecting affects less than 0.4% of the EU population between the ages of 15–64 but is associated with multiple health problems and social deprivation. Of major concern is the fact that opiate injectors have mortality rates 20 times higher than the general population due to overdoses, suicides, drug related illnesses and accidents. Injecting is the most common denominator of the most serious drug related health damage, potentially leading to the human immune-deficiency virus (HIV), the Hepatitis B virus (HBV) and the Hepatitis C virus (HCV). All three of these viruses are referred to as blood-borne viruses because of being transmitted via parenteral means. Russell and Carruthers (2005) give a detailed outline of the behaviours that put injecting drug users at risk and the issues that arise in attempting to undertake medical and psychosocial interventions for their prevention. Essentially the risks of becoming exposed to these viruses come from the sharing of needles and syringes, as well as other associated equipment such as cookers, cotton or water, and the blood to blood contact arising from giving or receiving injections. It is argued by Russell and Carruthers (2005: 368) that the common strategies used to deal with these common risk factors would be effective in tackling all three viruses, but in fact this is not the case; they make the point that these viruses 'differ in their prevalence and incidence among IDUs, their characteristics, natural histories and routes of transmission in ways that render generic prevention strategies inadequate'.

In terms of transmission HBV and HBC are easier to transmit than HIV through needle stick injuries. However, once infected, infection is chronic in all HIV cases but in 75–80% of HCV cases and in only 2–6% of HBV cases. Russell and Carruthers show that HIV rates in injecting drug users are variable whereas HBV and HCV infection are high for both viruses, but that a much higher proportion of HCV infections become chronic meaning that those who share injecting equipment are far more likely to come into contact with HCV than HBV. Another issue is that HBV, similar to HIV, is far more likely to be transmitted sexually, whereas HCV is rarely transmitted in this way. For all three viruses the only one for which there is an effective vaccination is HBV and this is an important approach to preventing its transmission.

Needle exchange is: 'The distribution of sterile injecting equipment and somewhere to dispose safely of used equipment in the form of needle exchange schemes, and has become a major approach to managing problem drug use' (Sheridan, 2005: 145). Needle exchange services, which distribute and dispose of needles, syringes and other injecting equipment (such as spoons, filters and citric acid), also typically offer advice and support on injecting more safely, injecting less, and preventing other people from starting to inject. These schemes will give advice and information on preventing infections associated with drug misuse, particularly HAV, HBV, HCV, and HIV. Importantly needle exchange schemes can act as a gateway to other services such as testing, advice, information and counselling around hepatitis and HIV vaccination for HAV and HBV and access to treatment for hepatitis HBV, HCV and HIV infection. Schemes will also offer advice and support on preventing overdose and drug related death as well as assessing clients and referring them to other treatment services if necessary. Drucker et al., (1998) found that harm reduction initiatives reduced the levels of HIV infection and AIDS and cut the frequency of heroin injection and the sharing of injecting equipment. These initiatives also have an impact upon the occurrence of sex work to buy drugs as well as the development of social skills and improvements in relationships.

Substitution treatment

Substitution treatment is a form of medical care offered to opiate addicts (primarily heroin addicts, but also amphetamine users (see below)) based on a similar or identical substance to the drug normally used. The use of substitute medications is part of an increasing range of pharmacological interventions intended to reduce the risk of harms associated with problematic drug use. It is estimated that there are 500,000 people across the world receiving substitute treatment, with 110,000 in the USA and 300,000 in Europe (2002). Substitute prescribing has two main aims: firstly, to impact upon adverse health and social outcomes, and secondly, to prescribe in a way that is safe for the individual and the community. Substitute treatment is now widespread across the European Union and a substantial consensus exists on its benefits, but it is not without controversy (Solberg et al., 2002). As with the term 'harm reduction' so with 'substitute prescribing' in that Farrell and Raistrick (2005) suggest that the terminology is imprecise and sometimes misleading. They argue that these programmes are driven by one of two major objectives namely, either to support health or social policy on the one hand and individual treatment on the other. They also suggest that very often these come into conflict as low threshold programmes and methadone maintenance are used to meet the first objective and methadone reduction the latter. Low threshold programmes have more or less open access and prescribe on demand, with this approach being associated with the Netherlands. These programmes are not used in the UK, but within the Dutch context are seen as being suitable for drug users who are unwilling or incapable of stopping their drug use and are assisted in reducing the harm associated with that use. Methadone reduction programmes are typically used in primary care settings in the UK, have a harm reduction goal, and are tailored towards achieving abstinence. Methadone maintenance has harm reduction aims and individuals typically move to this after unsuccessful attempts at reduction and abstinence.

In the UK the Department of Health's (1999) Clinical Guidelines in respect of substitute prescribing aim, firstly, to assist the patient in remaining healthy until they can achieve a drug free life; secondly, to reduce the use of illicit or non-prescribed drugs by the individual; thirdly, to deal with problems related to drug misuse; and fourthly, to reduce the dangers associated with drug misuse particularly in relation to blood-borne viruses and other infections arising from injecting and sharing injecting paraphernalia.

It has been argued that as amphetamine users are not usually physically dependent upon the drug then substitute prescribing is not appropriate. However, Fleming (2005) argues that the concept of an Amphetamine Dependence Syndrome is included in *DSM-IV* (American Psychiatric Association, 1994), including the broad criteria outlined in the previous chapter of increased salience, compulsion to use, tolerance and withdrawal symptoms. These symptoms can include listlessness, depression and sleepiness as well as craving, dysphoria, agitation, irritability and sleep disturbance. Fleming (2005) demonstrates that chronic amphetamine users frequently inject the drug and consequently experience a range of physical and psychological problems, very often not accessing services as these have traditionally been directed at opiate users.

There is plenty of evidence to show that substitute prescribing can reduce criminality, infectious diseases and drug related deaths, as well as improve the physical, psychological and social well-being of dependent users. There are, though, arguments that this approach fails to provide a real solution to drug, problems, creates a dependency upon another drug, and leads to crime insofar as the use of illicit methadone is a major problem. Some of these issues are addressed in the Scottish Government's new (2008) approach, which seeks to redress the balance that has seen such a huge move towards substitute prescribing, which is cheap and allows the UK government to more than meet its performance targets for the increasing numbers of people in treatment. However this approach may reduce choice, with people remaining on maintenance scripts rather than being given the option of more expensive longer term residential facilities to become drug free.

What are the substitute drugs?

Given that these approaches are contested amongst professionals and service users, a review of the acceptability and availability of pharmacological interventions in the UK was carried out by Rosenberg et al. (2002). They found that medications such as methadone, and Lofexidine for opiate users, substitute Benzodiazepines for Benzodiazepine dependence, Naltrexone for opiate relapse prevention, and Acamprosate for alcohol relapse prevention, were widely used and available. Other medications such as Buprenorphine for opiate detoxification, take home Naloxone for overdose prevention, and the substitute prescribing of levo-alpha-acetyl-methadol (LAAM), heroin and Dexamphetamine, although seen as acceptable approaches, were less popular.

Within the European Union over 90% of substitute prescribing is with methadone, with the rest using Buprenorphine which does not carry a risk of overdose and inhibits the parallel use of heroin. Methadone is very cheap to produce (Euro 8 per person per week), as compared with Buprenorphine (Euro 65 per person per week). Buprenorphine is preferred for some groups, for example pregnant women (Solberg et al., 2002).

It is argued by Anglin et al. (2007) that LAAM has some superior qualities to methadone in several important areas, including a reduction in positive tests for opiate use, the effective relief of withdrawal symptoms, as well as treatment retention. Like methadone, LAAM suppresses the withdrawal symptoms and blocks the intoxicating effects of opiate use; however, it has one other distinct and practical advantage over methadone in that it only needs to be administered three times weekly as opposed to daily. Additionally, methadone has variable effects on different people and is readily diverted into the black market.

Despite these issues with methadone (including the risk of overdose (see below)) the estimated number of drug users on methadone increased sixfold between 1993 and 1997. A report by the NTA (2007) highlighted that over the previous ten years there had been a doubling of methadone prescribing, which had been supplemented in the previous three years by an increase in the availability of Buprenorphine. This report argued that the 'British System' had been based upon flexible clinician prescribing which had been curtailed by more recent policy initiatives such as the National Drug Strategy (Home Office, 1998; 2002; 2008) and the creation of the National Treatment Agency. It would appear that a more centralised approach to drug treatment, focused primarily on crime reduction, has led to a massive increase in substitute prescribing.

The UK has taken a very different approach to other countries by including injectable heroin and methadone amongst its substitute therapies for people who are heroin dependent (Zador, 2005). This prescribing of heroin had been the crucial defining feature of the 'British System' since the Rolleston Committee in 1926, but has declined in favour of methadone prescribing. The *British Medical Journal* reports that about 300 people in the UK are regularly prescribed heroin and that this practice is enjoying something of a revival (Sheldon, 2008). A multi-site trial conducted in London, Brighton and Darlington, called the Randomised Injecting Opioid Treatment Trial (RIOTT), has compared the outcomes from injectable heroin and methadone with those from orally consumed methadone. RIOTT is a randomised controlled trial which examines the role of injectable opiate treatment for the management of heroin dependence in patients not responding to conventional substitution maintenance treatment. Approximately 150 subjects (50 in each group) were followed up for six months, comparing outcomes across a range of measures, including drug use, injecting practices, measures of global health and psychosocial functioning, criminality, treatment retention, incremental cost effectiveness, and measures of client satisfaction.

The trial was targeted at entrenched heroin addicts who despite receiving oral methadone maintenance treatment were continuing to inject street heroin almost every day. All groups achieved good retention but there was better retention in the injectable heroin group (88%) compared to 81% in the injectable methadone group and 69% in the oral methadone group.

The primary outcome measure of the trial was reduced use or abstinence from 'street' heroin and there was a reduction in street heroin use amongst all three treatment groups at the six months' stage. However, the most significant reduction was seen in the injectable heroin group with three-quarters responding well with a substantial reduction in the use of street heroin and with approximately 60% of the total group remaining abstinent (that is by allowing for no more than two lapses in drug testing during a three month period). Almost 20% of the total group were totally abstinent from street heroin which is significant in a group for whom daily illicit use while in treatment was the norm. For the injectable methadone and oral methadone groups the reductions were less significant, with about a third using street heroin on a less regular basis (www.kingshealthpartners. org/khp/2009/09/15/untreatable-or-just-hard-to-treat/).

> Should substitute prescribing be seen as just another medication?

Community prescribing

Under New Labour's ten year Drug Strategy (Home Office, 1998; 2002; 2008) the government has sought to increase the role of shared care arrangements for drug users, primarily with the involvement of GPs and nurses. In particular the Department of Health is committed to developing the nurse prescribing agenda by which nurses can prescribe, supply and administer medication. The stated aims of these approaches are 'designed to improve patients' access to medicines, develop workforce capacity, utilise skills more effectively and ensure the provision of more effective and accessible patient care' (National Treatment Agency, 2005: 1).

Community prescribing should be seen as a specialised drug treatment in the context of a care plan. It is provided as part of primary care, by a GP with an interest in drug misuse (shared care arrangements including under the auspices of a nurse prescriber) or by a doctor in a specialist drug treatment service, such as a Community Drug Team. Where clients receive the treatment may depend on the seriousness of their problems, how long they have been in treatment, or how stable they are. Community prescribing can include:

- stabilising a client on substitute drugs
- prescribing substitute drugs, such as methadone and Buprenorphine, for a sustained period (maintenance prescribing)
- prescribing for withdrawal (community detoxification)
- prescribing to prevent relapse
- stabilisation and withdrawal from sedatives, such as Valium and Temazepam
- prescribing for assisted withdrawal from alcohol, where appropriate
- treatment for stimulant users, which may include prescribing to help relieve symptoms
- non-medical prescribing (by nurses or pharmacists).

Research indicates that the dose of substitute given needs to match the former drug use level. It is offered in two forms: firstly, maintenance doses which prescribe enough substance to reduce risky or harmful behaviour; and secondly, gradually cutting the substance to zero (detox). Treatment comes with or without psychosocial support but it is recommended that additional support will lead to better outcomes from the treatment (EMCCDA, 2002). It is recognised that in determining the appropriate level of drug to prescribe that there is a process of negotiation between the staff and the service user (Quirk et al., 2003). This negotiation will address issues regarding the start dose and client perspectives on the amount of control allowed over changes to the dose, particularly any concerns over becoming addicted to methadone. Quirk et al. (2003) note that methadone has different meanings for different people, which shapes their goals in receiving a script, and this may in turn help to explain, for example, continued heroin use whilst on a methadone script.

CASE EXAMPLE

Whilst working as a manager the author, in partnership with a Community Alcohol and Drug Team (CADT), established a residential facility for detoxification from opiates. The protocol that was established was that the CADT would work

(Continued)

(Continued)

with a drug user to stabilise them on a methadone script and then reduce that dose to 25 Mg of methadone. At this point they would be admitted to the residential unit and placed on a Lofexidine script which would initially run concurrently with the methadone for 2/3 days before the methadone was halted all together and the course of Lofexidine completed over a 14 day period. This left the individual completely free of both the illicit drug and the substitute prescription, and would them allow them to enter a rehabilitation programme.

This example also highlights the need to try and work flexibly with the drug user to try and ensure the establishment of a meaningful and helping relationship. A 'focus on [the] everyday, lived experience' (Moore, 2005: 434) of drug users allows us an insight into the complexities of drug users' lives and a focus upon the service user also allows us to challenge some of the ideas that appear as received wisdom. In respect of clinical practice Dingwall et al. (1998, cited in Quirk et al., 2004: 41) argue that there are two aspects, namely the rules that emerge from the evidence based upon randomised controlled trials and the ways in which practitioners improvise in using the general skills for a particular case. The development of the National Treatment Agency and a centralised approach to addressing drug issues have also seen a major impetus to achieving a service user perspective on the development of practice, in that 'The NTA wants to build an equal partnership with treatment service users and drug users, because … we respect the unique expertise and experiences of users and understand the health, esteem and other personal benefits that involvement can bring' (www.nta.nhs.uk/areas/users_and_carers/user_involvement.aspx).

> What are the implications of this quote for practitioners given that the drug use being referred to is a criminal offence?

Mortality amongst drug users

In terms of mortality amongst drug users other than disease there are three main areas to be considered, namely overdose, suicide and trauma (Darke et al., 2007). Darke et al. show that there is a completed suicide risk 14 times that of the general population for people with an opiate dependence, but also four times the risk for cannabis dependence, 45 times for Benzodiazepine dependence and six times for alcohol dependence. In addition, dependent drug users are far more likely to be suffering from Post Traumatic Stress Disorder, particularly as life threatening events and serious physical assault appear to be very common amongst opiate users. However, overdose is the primary cause of death amongst injecting drug users across Europe, Australia and the USA (Hickman et al., 2003; Seymour et al., 2003), but is substantially lower for those on methadone maintenance programmes (Brugal et al., 2005). There is conclusive evidence to show that the risk of overdose appears to increase following periods of relative abstinence due to detoxification, rehabilitation, or imprisonment (Hickman et al., 2008), and that overdose increases dramatically in the first month after a discharge from treatment (Davoli et al., 2007). The reasons for overdose are complex but typically involve the combined use of opiates and particularly depressant drugs such as alcohol and Benzodiazepines, with overdose from heroin alone being very rare (National Treatment Agency, nd). Whilst it is argued by Darke (2008) that this should come as no surprise and in fact, given the nature of drugs that suppress the central nervous system, it would be astonishing if they were not implicated, others (Hickman et al., 2008) have speculated that the relationship is not such a simple one.

Hickman et al. (2008) reviewed the prevailing theories of the causes of overdose which include the view that alcohol and opiates (particularly heroin) have additive or interactive pharmacological effects on depressing respiration, so that if alcohol is consumed then less heroin is required to induce overdose. However, it is also possible that alcohol consumption distorts the user's judgement as to their tolerance and safe amounts to use. Heroin users who are abstaining or cutting down may drink more alcohol, and in this case a reducing heroin tolerance may be the issue rather than a specific effect of alcohol. For those in treatment it has been found that about one-third of people on methadone drink alcohol excessively (Senbanjo et al., 2006) and NTORS (Gossop et al., 2003) found that, whilst there were improvements across the problem domains, this was not the case for alcohol consumption. This may be because programmes which are focused on illicit drug use have not prioritised the use of a legal substance and, for example, may view it in the same way as smoking tobacco. This has led Senbanjo et al. (2006) amongst others to argue that treatment providers need to adopt interventions that will address the full range of alcohol problems and supplementary services for multiple needs. Hickman et al. (2008) also suggest that poly drug use may be a feature of people with an increased risk of overdose for broader psychological and social reasons. This is supported by Darke (2008) who points to evidence that the majority of overdoses, both fatal and non-fatal, occur in familiar surroundings and amongst a population with high levels of psychopathology as well as serious health problems.

The UK Government introduced a three-year action plan to reduce drug related deaths in 2001 which set a target of a 20% reduction in drug related deaths by March 2004. This would represent about 300 lives saved nationally and many of these deaths would be easily preventable. However, it is obvious that HIV and hepatitis infections have the capacity to cause far more deaths in the future, therefore the NTA (nd) argues that there needs to be an approach that addresses both short and long term issues. However, the evaluation of this approach demonstrated that deaths were not reduced by as many as had been intended and that the rate of blood-borne virus infection may be rising (NTA/DoH, 2008). A new action plan was launched in 2007 which attempted to take an integrated approach at national, regional, and local levels. The key aspects of this strategy are the benchmarking all local drug partnerships in terms of the commissioning and provisioning of harm reduction services, the development and implementation of local action plans to improve harm reduction in the poorest performing areas identified in the service review, and for all local drug partnerships to work with regional NTA teams to address specific harm reduction issues identified in the service review.

Most overdoses occur in the presence of other people, often other drug users who may be reluctant to call the medical services due to the fear of police involvement. Consequently one of the approaches that has been developed is the training of drug users themselves in overdose prevention strategies, so that they can identify and respond to incidents of overdose. Naloxone is a drug that can be administered via injection to quickly and safely reverse the effects of overdose. In New York over a one-year period over 1000 participants were trained in Skills and Knowledge in Opiate Prevention (SKOOP) and were given a prescription for Naloxone by a medical doctor attending a needle exchange scheme. A review of the scheme has been carried out by Piper et al. (2007). Opiate users were trained either individually, in pairs, or in small groups, with the teaching and discussion centring around the following curriculum: the causes of opiate overdose, how to avoid an overdose, and signs of an opiate overdose. Information was given about: Naloxone; education about appropriate responses to overdose, such as calling medical services and performing rescue breathing; the administration of Naloxone through intra-muscular injection; and the possible need for a second dose of the drug. The finding of Piper et al. (2007) supported by other studies is that the use of Naloxone distribution and the training of opiate users in overdose prevention work is effective in reducing deaths from overdose. This approach is used in the UK and also with the recommendation that all workers who come into contact with people at risk of overdose are trained in the administration of Naloxone.

Conclusion

Harm reduction approaches have become a major feature of the international agenda to reduce the risk of harm associated with (primarily but not exclusively) injecting drug use. Although these approaches lack clarity in terms of definition and clinical practice there is plenty of evidence to demonstrate their effectiveness in reducing a range of medical, psychological, and social harms. In addition, substitutes such as methadone are cheap to produce and enable a relatively 'easy' definition of 'treatment', which allows practitioners and commissioners to demonstrate that they are meeting their targets for getting people into treatment. It should come as no surprise that, within the UK context, the New Labour target of increasing the number of people in treatment by 100% between 1998 and 2008 was accompanied by a huge increase in the use of methadone. Just as ethical considerations give rise to the need for harm reduction approaches to effectively help drug users, so the outcomes from those approaches raise their own set of issues in terms of drug users having choice around treatment modalities, becoming completely drug free, and receiving adequate psychosocial interventions.

Useful resources

Drugscope – www.drugscope.org.uk/
National Treatment Agency for Substance Misuse – www.nta.nhs.uk/
The Methadone Alliance – www.m-alliance.org.uk/

5

The Psychological Revolution

The aims of this chapter are to:

- consider the developments in cognitive and behavioural approaches to understanding addiction
- consider the impact of ideas that have informed harm minimisation and controlled drinking approaches, and the development of social learning techniques
- pay particular attention to the core psychological constructs of motivation, self-efficacy, and self-esteem
- discuss issues of co-morbidity.

Psychology has been instrumental in analysing the dimensional nature of addiction and in helping the move away from the unitary disease perspective. Heather and Robertson (1997) describe this as a 'paradigm shift'. In practice this shift in thinking has been a difficult and contentious one that has challenged the orthodoxy of irreversibility, pathology, and abstinence as the only realistic goal that the 'alcoholic' or 'addict' should be aiming towards. Of huge importance has been the realisation that drug use exists on a continuum with the possibility of people moving in and out of problems and dependence over the course of time (see Heather and Robertson, 1997). This has not only led to improvements in public health approaches but has also meant increased interest in a number of inter-linked areas such as relapse prevention, relapse management, harm reduction, and controlled drug use. The latter has particularly been associated with the alcohol field whereby the issue of 'controlled drinking' has stirred real debate in terms of its ethical basis and efficacy (Heather and Robertson, 1981).

In the field of substance misuse, and particularly in relation to treatments, psychological approaches can be divided into three broad areas: learning theory based models, psychodynamic theories, and transtheoretical models (Wanigaratne, 2006), with most interventions being based on cognitive and behavioural theories (Curran and Drummond, 2007). In this chapter we will review the main psychological models utilised in the field of addiction influenced by learning theories and transtheoretical approaches. The key issues arising from psychodynamic theories as 'talking therapies', namely the importance of establishing therapeutic and empathic relationships, will be explored in Chapters 7 and 8.

The psychological principles that have been applied to alcohol misuse are reviewed by Heather and Robertson (1981) who point out that a unified theory does not exist in this area and that different psychological principles have been applied to different facets of addiction. They use the examples of classical conditioning theory being applied to explain craving and cognitive approaches for relapse. Whilst some researchers have sought a unified theory (notably Orford's (2002) excessive appetites modes and West's (2006) PRIME theory (see below)), the key principles of learning by an individual interacting with their environment remain, through the processes of classical conditioning, operant conditioning, skilled behaviour, self-control, and cognitive learning. This conditioning is caused by external environmental cues, the rewards associated with the drug taking behaviour, and an inability neither to regulate drug use nor to recognise situations which are perpetuating the drug use, as well as distorted thinking around the drug use (Heather and Robertson, 1981).

It is important to realise that much of our conditioning occurs at a level of which we are not conscious so that thoughts and actions become routine within particular contexts and automatic, with the neurobiology of the brain's own reward mechanisms having an essential part to play in this process (see Chapter 6 on neurobiology).

> How aware are you of your habits and rituals? To what extent do you do them automatically without 'thinking' about them, for example having a cigarette, or an alcoholic drink, or a cup of tea/coffee, at particular times and in particular settings?

Interests in the principles of learning and the commonalities across different problem areas are central to Social Learning Theory. This theory is concerned with how human behaviour is acquired, maintained, and changed (Lindstrom, 1992), irrespective of whether it is viewed as 'normal' or 'deviant'. It is argued that this behaviour can be identified, measured, and altered through an understanding of antecedent cues, reinforcing the consequences, modelling, and expectancies from the behaviour. Lindstrom (1992) and West (2006) outline the core assumptions of this approach, arguing that no behaviour is simple enough to be acquired by a single learning mechanism but that there are contingencies that will reinforce drug use and dependence. These contingencies are the positive reinforcement associated with the taking of a substance, such as euphoria and relaxation; the positive reinforcement of the social aspects of drug use; the negative reinforcement associated with some aversive environmental or psychological aspects, such as boredom or an escape from unpleasant living conditions; a negative reinforcement related to aversive physical states, such as the avoidance of withdrawal symptoms or a relief of pain; and a negative reinforcement related to attempts to alter psychological states such as anxiety.

As well as behavioural processes, cognitive psychology has also made a huge contribution to our understanding of addiction. Although there are different approaches within this discipline, Eysenck (1993) argues that the primary subject matters are the processes of attention, perception, learning, memory, language, concept formation, problem solving, and thinking. The use of cognitive psychology in addressing substance misuse has been particularly influential via the work of Marlatt and Gordon (1985, see below) and their study of relapse prevention. This model and the work of DiClemente and Prochaska (1998) are built around the core constructs of motivation and self-efficacy. Additionally, and in relation to concepts of identity, self-esteem is an important issue. It is important to note that these psychological processes apply to all human beings in all situations, and so in line with the psychological processes outlined above they seek to explain addiction within the context of general human behaviour.

In understanding these issues within a context of general human behaviour and within a biopsychosocial framework, insights are then gained from looking at a range of behaviours that may be addictive. Orford (2002), in developing his model of Excessive Appetites, reviews drinking, gambling, drug taking, eating, exercising, and sexual behaviour, and argues that the 'development of desires and inclinations–appetites is basic to life' (2002: 1). In this sense addiction can arise out of any behaviour and Orford explains the process of addiction by looking at the ways in which a behaviour is taken up and the individual factors that may contribute to it; the ways in which restraint may be overcome and a strong attachment to the behaviour developed; the role of internal conflict or ambivalence about the behaviour; and the roles of decision making and self-control.

One of the key models used in practice to analyse and change problematic behaviour is the Trans-Theoretical Model of Change (TTM) (DiClemente and Prochaska, 1998) which is a complex three dimensional model comprising stages, processes, and levels of change that has become ubiquitous in professional practice. The TTM is not in itself a theory of addiction, but a model of intentional behavioural change. Although the TTM has been heavily critiqued (particularly by West, 2006), for our purposes the model is an attempt to identify the core components of behavioural change that can be identified by reviewing the outcome literature on a range of therapeutic interventions, including cognitive, behavioural, humanistic, and existential approaches. The TTM incorporates the psychological constructs of self-efficacy and motivation and allows us to consider these processes in more detail. The model has been applied across a wide range of disciplines including approaches to dealing with tobacco use, illicit drug use, alcohol use, weight control, exercise, eating disorders, mental health, child welfare, domestic violence, organisational change, psychotherapy, and offender rehabilitation.

DiClemente and Prochaska (1998) argue that a truly comprehensive model of behavioural change must not only be applicable across a range of addictive behaviours, but also must address the spectrum of ways in which people change. This spectrum covers self-help, to brief interventions, through to intensive therapeutic interventions; different people may need different approaches at different times. An aim of the TTM is to try and synthesise diverse treatment methods, by searching for core processes of behavioural change. This search for core processes from diverse approaches is consistent with the psychological argument proposed by Bandura (1977) that all behaviours stem from common causes. This is supported by Orford (2008: 879) who argues that 'there is increasing support for the existence of important change processes that are common to treatments with different names and theoretical rationales'.

The Trans-Theoretical Model of Change (TTM)

Stages of change

The stages of change are also known as the Cycle of Change and 'represent the dynamic and motivational aspects of the process of change over time' (DiClemente and Prochaska, 1998: 4). It is argued that the stages represent the specific tasks required to achieve a successful and sustained behavioural change. The authors of the model argue that five stages have been successfully identified:

1 Pre-contemplation – an individual is unaware that they have a problem, or are aware but do not want to do anything about it within the next six months.
2 Contemplation – the individual is starting to think seriously about change and is weighing up the pros and cons of making that change within the next six months. They may move forward, or not, and ambivalence is normal at this stage.
3 Preparation – the individual makes the decision to change and makes a commitment to the change being implemented in the next month.
4 Action – the planned behavioural change is implemented and active coping is initiated. This stage may last for between one and six months.
5 Maintenance – if the action stage lasts for between three and six months then the individual moves into the maintenance stage whereby the change must become fully integrated into the lifestyle.

In addition a new 'termination' stage has been added in which the individual has fully adopted the new behaviour pattern (West, 2006).

Working with relapse

To what extent should we view relapse as a failure on the part of an individual?

Within the work of Marlatt and Gordon (1985) and that of Prochaska and DiClemente (1982), relapse is seen as a process that develops over the course of time starting before the initial use of a substance and continuing once that substance has been consumed. Importantly, Marlatt and Gordon develop a social aspect to their model and identify the importance of environmental factors in leading to relapse. They identify incidences which situationally may determine relapse which include: intrapersonal negative emotional states such as anger, anxiety, depression, frustration and boredom; interpersonal conflicts with family and friends; and social pressure of both a direct and indirect kind and positive emotional states such as celebrations.

Relapse is identified within the TTM with the understanding that, within addictive behaviours, it is the norm rather than the exception. In the research by Prochaska and DiClemente (1982) they found that people would revolve around the cycle of change on average between six and eight times before giving up smoking. In diagrammatic representations of the cycle, relapse is also usually shown as a stage, with the implication being that individuals will move back into the pre-contemplation stage. This cyclical model has clear links with social learning theory and raises new possibilities for interventions that might consider not just relapse prevention approaches but also relapse management in terms of continuing with appropriate interventions.

How might harm reduction approaches help in managing relapse?

The importance of this cannot be overstated because the notion of relapse management is in complete contradistinction to popular disease models utilised by Alcoholics Anonymous and Narcotics Anonymous. Whilst the Twelve Step disease model agrees with the idea of impaired control, it also argues that alcoholics or addicts have an abnormal craving for drugs which marks them out from other people. The principles of social learning theory are that anybody can develop problematic behaviour or become addicted to drugs, whereas the Twelve Step view is that alcoholics and addicts are physically and mentally different to the rest of the population. However, in terms of interventions the psychological approach has highlighted a major problem with the goal of total abstinence which is the abstinence violation effect (AVE). In practice this may mean either stopping completely or cutting down (a harm minimisation or controlled drinking approach), but, whichever goal is aimed for, it is still a matter of control. However, when trying for complete abstinence and engaging in initial use of a drug (a slip or lapse) then feelings of failure, guilt and anger may ensue which lead to continued drug use so that a full relapse occurs. People who use AA say 'that one drink is too many and a thousand is not enough'. Relapse management tries to teach control mechanisms so that drug use does not increase, thereby maintaining the viability of the original goal. Within this approach and as it is expressed within the TTM, a mature understanding of relapse would view lapse and relapse as opportunities to review what is and is not working in achieving personal treatment goals.

Processes of change

These processes are seen as 'the engines that facilitate movement through the stages of change' (DiClemente and Prochaska, 1998: 4) and are derived from diverse therapeutic approaches. Ten of these processes have been identified which relate to particular stages of change:

1 Consciousness raising is concerned with the drug user becoming aware of their drug use and the consequences of that use and the reasons why the drug use continues.
2 Self-liberation reflects an increase in self-efficacy with the belief that change and the achievement of desirable goals are possible.
3 Social liberation involves environmental changes which may include a new job, or mixing with non-drug using peers.

4   Counter-conditioning is the use of cognitive and behavioural techniques to identify and overcome conditioned responses such as drinking in particular situations with particular people or on the basis of particular feelings.

5   Stimulus control seeks to restructure the environment from which the drug taking cues arise (classical conditioning). This may involve avoiding certain places, situations or people.

6   Self-re-evaluation is the process whereby the drug user realises that their drug taking is in conflict with their sense of self or longer term goals in life. This involves a weighing up of the pros and cons of change.

7   Social re-evaluation considers the same aspects but in respect of other people who may be being affected by the drug use.

8   Contingency management looks to the consequences of drug taking rather than its antecedents, and seeks to find ways of rewarding positive changes in drug taking behaviour or punishing negative changes.

9   Dramatic relief refers to change via a cathartic experience or insight into one's behaviour.

10   Helping relationship refers to any relationship professional, non-professional or informal that assists in the motivation to change.

The TTM provides a psychological framework for interventions that are informed by a range of insights from behavioural and cognitive psychology. In addition these processes can be divided into those which are experiential and those which are behavioural. This distinction is important because it is one thing to think about doing something and another to actually do it. Traditional psychoanalysis based on the work of Freud and Jung was predicated upon the concept of abreaction, whereby the repressed emotions caused by trauma are expressed and the catharsis gives way to behavioural change (Yalom, 1980). However, studies have found that these traditional approaches are not effective in leading to behavioural change in contrast to cognitive and behavioural approaches (see Miller et al., 1998).

Levels of change

The third part of the TTM involves the levels of change which recognise that addictive behaviours often have multiple problem areas that interact with each other. DiClemente and Prochaska (1998) recognise that individuals may be in different stages of change with respect to different problem areas. Psychology recognises the importance of the individual in context and the influences that those contexts and the individuals concerned have upon each other (Gifford and Humphreys, 2007). These levels of change have received very little attention within either the practitioner or academic communities but may in fact represent an important shift to a more systems and a complexity orientated understanding of addiction. This is interesting because the levels of change start to address the issues of multiple needs in the form of poly drug use, concurrent mental health problems, and the range of social and environmental deficits identified by NTORS (Gossop et al., 1998), as well as the other international longitudinal studies (see Chapter 1).

There is a need for theory building in this area and the levels of change, whilst not fully developing these ideas, move us in the direction of mutually reinforcing factors that need to be addressed in understanding and working with addiction. The levels identified by DiClemente and Prochaska are as follows and go from the most superficial to the most profound:

Symptom/situational in which the primary concern is to change the behaviour and its antecedents. For example, a person may be experiencing work related stress and anxiety and so is drinking alcohol to try and alleviate that stress. An approach would be to deal with the work situation either by trying to manage the tasks differently or to recognise that taking another job is a desirable outcome.

Maladaptive cognitions are the automatic or unconscious thoughts that maintain behaviour. The person managing stress through drinking may be unaware that they are having negative thoughts about their ability to deal with these situations.

Interpersonal conflicts and family/systems conflict refer to areas that are major causes of relapse (Marlatt and Gordon, 1985) due to conflict with family and friends. Anecdotally, when I worked with people with substance misuse problems one of the biggest causes of relapse was due to dealing with the Department of Social Security to claim state benefits. Traditional psychotherapeutic approaches also acknowledge the family as the primary cause of behavioural problems (Yalom, 2005).

Intrapersonal conflicts refer to long-standing internal conflicts that cause an individual's identity to be bound up with their behaviour; they may see themselves as an addict or an alcoholic in a pathological way. In addition, there is a strong association between traumatic experiences, such as experiencing childhood abuse, and substance misuse. There is debate as to whether it is necessary to try and resolve the issues that have caused the trauma before a positive outcome for addiction treatment can be experienced (Fiorentine, 1998). These issues have an impact on the sense of self and have clear links with the concept of self-esteem (see below).

Motivation

Miller (2006: 134) argues that 'addiction is fundamentally a problem of motivation', but importantly that this is not the same as saying that it is simply the result of people being unmotivated to address problematic behaviour and therefore worthy of moral blame. Along with West (2001; 2006) and Koob (2006), Miller links the psychology of motivation to the neuro-scientific understanding of the brain's reward systems. Within the biopsychosocial paradigm it is important not to privilege biology over the other factors (Orford 2002) and there are obviously complex connections here between biology, context, and the expectancies of individuals using drugs (see Edwards, 2004). The issue of motivation is at the heart of Motivational Interviewing (MI) that has been developed by Miller and Rollnick (2002) as a key adjunct to the cycle of change. Along with the TTM, MI has also become a key feature of professional services. (See Chapter 7 for a discussion of the importance of motivational working.)

Self-efficacy

Self-efficacy has been presented by Bandura (1977) as a unifying theory of behaviour and 'plays a unique role in the addictive behaviours field ... [influencing] both the initial development of addictive habits and the behaviour change process' (Marlatt et al., 1995: 289). Self-efficacy is a core construct within cognitive and behavioural approaches and also a key part of the TTM. Bandura (1977) defines self-efficacy as the belief on the part of an individual that they can cope with a situation which is of high risk to them in terms of engaging in unwanted behaviour. This is particularly relevant to addiction whereby certain situations may increase the risk of relapse and there is a substantial body of literature linking the development of self-efficacy with positive treatment outcomes (see Marlatt et al., 1995). Marlatt and Gordon's (1985) relapse prevention model posits the idea that an individual with coping skills, when faced with a high risk situation, is more likely to be able to deal with that situation in a functional way that in itself leads to an increase in confidence. Self-efficacy can be seen as a positive feedback loop which is linked to notions of mastery over our own personal environments (Dweck, 2000). In dealing with addictions it has been identified that it is success and trying to be successful that eventually predict success (Westerberg, 1998). Conversely, a failure to succeed can lead to an increased risk of relapse and an increased salience of drug taking behaviour.

In practice Bandura's theory of self-efficacy is somewhat narrow in focus, partly because he makes a clear distinction between it and the other self concept of self-esteem. Bandura (1977) argues that there is a difference between the two concepts because it is quite possible to achieve personal goals, aims, and objectives without having a sense of self-worth or feeling good about it. There is no doubt form the research that self-efficacy (based upon situational confidence) is important precisely because it varies from situation to situation for individuals. However, this narrow definition of self-efficacy feeds into the TTM which does not therefore identify concepts related to self-esteem. A consequence of this may be that our ability to theorise about and work with individuals who have the most complex problems may be hampered because of important links between confidence, self-worth, and identify which will be discussed below.

> Identify some situations in which you are confident and feel in control, and some where the opposite is true.

Self-esteem

There are a number of differing definitions of self-esteem and a comprehensive account of these and their components is provided by Mruk (1999), while Emler (2001) supplies a good overview of the causes and consequences of low self-esteem. Mruk (1999) identifies that self-esteem is linked to identity and behaviour, and that positive self-esteem correlates with positive mental health and psychological well-being, whereas low self-esteem is correlated with depression and a range of other mental health disorders, as well as a lack of adequate personal and social functioning. The key to Bandura's view of the differences between self-esteem and self-efficacy lies in the relationship between confidence and feelings of worthiness. However, as Mruk (1999) identifies there are a number of differing definitions of self-esteem which incorporate differing components, and probably the one most widely used is the Rosenberg Self Esteem Scale (Emler, 2001) which emphasises worthiness.

However, other definitions consider other dimensions to self-esteem such as confidence (competence), cognition as well as feelings, stability and openness. Whereas self-efficacy is seen as being situational and relatively open to change, self-esteem is seen as stabilising in late adolescence and whilst it may fluctuate will return to a general level. A reading of Mruk will indicate that a mature definition of self-esteem which incorporates other components may provide us with opportunities to develop our work with individuals who engage in problematic behaviour.

The third dimension of the TTM are the levels of change in which DiClemente and Prochaska (1998) identify that individuals' problematic behaviour may affect different areas of their lives to the point that they may experience intrapsychic conflict so that their sense of self or identity is bound up with that behaviour. This process of social, professional or self-labelling, which designates someone as an 'alcoholic', 'junkie', or 'piss head', indicates a strong link with 'self esteem [which] is central to the dynamics of the identity process' (Breakwell and Rowett, 1982). These issues concerning identity are often bound up with multiple problem areas, and at a time when people are presenting to services with increasingly complex matrices of problems, including poly drug use, homelessness, mental and physical health problems, and offending behaviour amongst others (see Gossop et al., 2003), then this is an important area for theory building to inform effective practice. The levels of change are an important but ultimately limited attempt to address the issues related to identity and multiple needs. Given that 'psychology is the study of the individual in context' (Gifford and Humphreys, 2007: 352) these levels do not give sufficient attention to other factors particularly social ones which affect behaviour (Barber, 1995).

The study of psychology in context has given us models that reflect our increasing understanding of the complex nature of addiction and thus the need to address biopsychosociality. In addressing these issues and moving us towards an understanding of complexity theory itself (see Chapter 8) West (2006) has developed his PRIME theory of addiction.

For West, addiction defined as 'a behaviour over which an individual has impaired control with harmful consequences' (2001: 3) means that it affects an individual's capacity to make rational choices and thus is best viewed both as a psychiatric disorder and a disorder of motivation. West (2006: 147) outlines the five levels of the human motivational system (PRIME) which he argues are fundamental to addiction:

1   Plans (conscious mental representations of future action plus commitment).
2   Responses (starting, stopping, or modifying actions).
3   Impulses/inhibitory forces (can be consciously experienced as urges).
4   Motives (can be consciously experienced as desires).
5   Evaluations (evaluative beliefs).

An analytical approach to this would be the expectation that an individual plans to change a behaviour, undertakes the necessary actions, deals with urges, builds the motivation to maintain change and on the basis of evaluating the benefits experienced reinforces those changes. However, people do not always have the resources to makes changes; urges and cravings can be over-powering; changes can lead to negative emotional states; and the evaluation may lead to continued ambivalence. Any one of these levels can over-power the rest. West argues that within this system any one of the five levels can function abnormally, that all of the levels can interact together (to differing degrees), and that 'elements come into and out of existence as a result of influences within the system' (2006: 147). These interactions are dynamic and multi-dimensional in nature and due to their fundamental non-linearity do not allow for simple predictions of cause and effect.

Dual diagnosis

Within all of these models the issue of psychiatric distress is a major confounding and complicating set of problems, where the issue of 'dual diagnosis' is common and presents a real problem for practitioners, the commissioners of services, and policy makers. The terms 'dual diagnosis' and 'co-morbidity' are used interchangeably and are also used to describe the co-existence of one or more mental disorders in individuals who have a diagnosis of a substance use disorder, or vice versa (Todd et al., 2004). The terms usually denote severe mental illness and include psychosis, schizophrenia, bipolar affective illness, and substance use disorders. However there are critiques of this terminology, with the observation being made that this group of people is heterogeneous in nature, experiencing a multiplicity of needs rather than just two 'illnesses' (see Drake et al., 2004).

The concept of dual diagnosis first emerged in the 1980s with the advent of de-institutionalisation and 'care in the community'. When removed from the protective surroundings of institutional living, access to alcohol and drugs is increased along with the harms associated with that use (Mueser et al., 1998). Since then research into this area has consistently identified that the co-occurrence of the problems is common. For example, in the UK the National Psychiatric Morbidity surveys found a clear relationship between a dependence on nicotine, alcohol and drugs and psychiatric disorders (Meltzer, 1995). In the NTORS study of 1075 drug users entering treatment 10% had received hospital psychiatric treatment and 14% community psychiatric treatment for a problem other than drug dependence in the two years prior to intake (Gossop et al., 1998; see Chapter 1). According to the Department of Health, Community Mental Health Teams report that 8 to 15% of their service users have a dual diagnosis although this may be higher in some inner city areas. These high levels are found across the industrialised world; a study by Regier et al. (1990) which surveyed 19,000 individuals across the USA found a prevalence rate for substance use disorders of 16.7%. However, for people experiencing schizophrenia this increased to 47%, for affective disorders 32%, and for anxiety disorders 23.7%.

Other than the broad social, cultural and political issues involved in the process of de-institutionalisation there are a number of theories which seek to explain increased co-morbidity. These are reviewed by Mueser et al. (1998) who argue that no single model can account for all cases of dual diagnosis and that any one model can apply to any individual.

Common factor models

These models look at risk factors that are shared across both substance use and serious mental illness with particular reference to genetic factors and anti-social personality disorder. There is evidence to show that genetic factors contribute to schizophrenia, bi-polar disorder, and substance use disorders. It is argued by Mueser et al. that the heritability of schizophrenia and alcohol misuse does not account for increased rates of substance misuse amongst people with severe mental illness.

In the USA, Anti Social Personality Disorder (ASPD) has been the focus of much research, with the evidence suggesting that ASPD and Conduct Disorder (CD) are strongly linked to substance use disorders. As there is also strong evidence for a link between APSD and severe mental illness as well as the other two disorders there is a suggestion that APSD is a common factor between all of them. However, Mueser et al. critique the way that APSD is constructed with its emphasis on criminal behaviour and ignoring the context in which the behaviour emerges. Rather than describing a mental illness the ASPD construct may well be describing the consequences of social problems, poverty, and cognitive factors.

In terms of common factors, Mueser et al. argue that it is precisely these socio-economic factors based upon education, income, and occupation which are important in determining higher rates of both severe mental illness and substance misuse. Cognitive impairment also leads to increased risks for mental illness and substance misuse and Mueser et al. speculate that socio-economic status and cognitive impairment work in conjunction with other risk factors to contribute to co-morbidity.

Secondary substance use disorder models

These models argue that severe mental illness increases an individual's vulnerability to developing substance misuse disorders and that they fall into the two categories of psychosocial risk factor models and the biologically based super-sensitivity model. The psychosocial model focuses on the components of self-medication and the alleviation of dysphoria, as well as multiple risk factors. The self-medication perspective argues that individuals choose specific substances for their pharmacological properties within specific effects in specific situations. In the research literature there is little evidence to support this medicating approach although it is clear that individuals are aware of the effects of drugs and their reactions to them. Mueser et al. argue that self-report studies show that dually diagnosed people use substances to alleviate social problems, insomnia, depression, and other conditions that exist across diagnoses, but rarely to alleviate specific symptoms. Another important issue related to drug selection is that drug use is very much based upon availability and market forces.

CASE EXAMPLE

Sean is a man in his thirties, unemployed, living in hostels, and in and out of detox and rehab programmes. He has an addiction to alcohol and smokes tobacco and cannabis. He receives medication for depression and for psychotic symptoms, such as negative voices in his head that tell him to do 'bad things'. For Sean, sometimes the voices get so bad and persistent that the only way he can deal with them is to drink excessively, which gives him some short term relief. But he knows that the drinking will make the voices worse in the medium term.

More generally the alleviation of dysphoria is a model that looks to negative experiences such as anxiety, depression, boredom, and loneliness as drivers for substance use, rather than the specific approach of the self-medication hypothesis. The alleviation of dysphoria approach is also subsumed into the multiple risk factor model, with common risk factors including social isolation, poor interpersonal and cognitive skills, school and vocation failure, an association with deviant sub-groups, and living in areas with high availability of drugs.

The super sensitivity approach argues that a combination of genetic and early environmental events interacts with environmental stress to cause a psychiatric disorder. A compromised biological sensitivity to stress may also apply to the effects of psychoactive substances. This may explain why people with severe mental illness may experience more negative consequences from smaller amounts of drug use than people in the general population. This does not, however, explain all dual diagnoses across all psychiatric disorders and include all of the types of drug used.

Secondary psychiatric illness models

The assumption of this model is that substance use can lead to severe mental illness and is notably a feature of the current debates within the UK concerning the classification of cannabis. Debates have focused on the drugs that can mimic psychotic episodes such as stimulants and hallucinogens as well as cannabis (see the section on alcohol and cannabis).

Bi-directional models

These models suggest that there are interacting effects between substance use disorders and severe mental illness that can account for increased co-morbidity and this is a theme that will be developed in the chapter on complexity theory.

Conclusion

Psychology has made a significant contribution to the understanding of substance use and misuse. In particular it has identified core processes which are significant in learning and maintaining behaviours, which may well be harmful to the individuals concerned. These core processes have played an important part in developing interventions to address those problematic behaviours and have also highlighted the need to engage with both behaviour and cognitions in leading to positive outcomes. It is important to realise that these psychological processes are also directly linked to biological and social factors and, for the same reasons that biological factors are insufficient on their own, to address the issues of addiction, so too psychology. The issues associated with substance misuse and psychiatric co-morbidity demonstrate that the causes and consequences of addiction are multi-factorial in nature and require a more integrated approach to understanding and working with these.

Useful resources

MIND – www.mind.org.uk/

Miller, W. and Heather, N. (eds) (1998) *Treating Addictive Behaviors* (2nd edition). New York: Penum.

Orford, J. (2001) *Excessive Appetites: A Psychological View of Addictions*. Chichester: Wiley.

West, R. (2006) *Theory of Addiction*. Oxford: Blackwell Publishing.

6

The Genetic Revolution and Disease Theory Revisited

The aims of this chapter are to:

- review the idea of addiction as a disease through the lens of developments in the field of genetics, neurobiology and evolutionary theory
- consider the implications of these developments for our understanding of addiction
- consider these points with particular reference to an ethical basis for the nature of interventions.

Over the last 30 years there has been a revolution in our understanding of the basis and development of biological life, the workings of the brain, and the nature of consciousness itself. This revolution has had implications as much for our understanding of substance use and addiction as it has for other areas. The last three chapters have demonstrated that there has been in existence three broad models of addictive behaviour; the classical disease model being very much based upon the experiences of people who have addictions, the dependency syndromes based upon the clinical impressions of practitioners, and psychological approaches seeking a more evidence based perspective. Each approach has its strengths and weaknesses in terms of theory building and also in identifying the foundations for interventions, but in themselves would seem to leave some significant gaps in our knowledge base: the disease perspective does not allow for diversity in addictive experiences and ways of overcoming those problems; dependence syndromes appear to take a highly medicalised view with an emphasis on dependence as being a distinct phenomenon from problems; and conversely psychology does not give enough attention to some of the medico-biological issues. This polarisation of positions is most obviously seen in the range of interventions that is offered, with little cross fertilisation of ideas between Twelve Step Programmes, medical interventions such as detoxification, and cognitive-behavioural and psychotherapeutic approaches.

A number of critical advances have occurred that are interlinked and have started to give us new and profound insights into the nature of drug use and how this use can lead to a state of addiction; these advances are in neurobiology, the unravelling of the human genome, evolutionary theory, and the understanding of complex systems. This chapter will consider genetics and neurobiology within an evolutionary context and the ways in which they contribute to the biopsychosocial paradigm. In Chapter 8 we will consider complexity theory as a basis for understanding the kind of complex system that addiction constitutes. But in the first instance it is important to consider the building blocks of that system and in particular the advances in our understanding of biological functioning, together with the impact that psychoactive drugs have upon those mechanisms.

The evolutionary context

Since Charles Darwin published *On the Origin of Species* in 1859, our understanding of the ways in which evolution happens, and what this means for life in general, has developed exponentially. Increasingly this approach is being used to understand human behaviour and there is a growing body of literature which applies it to drug use and addiction and to the biopsychosocial paradigm (Lende and Smith, 2002). Evolution is primarily concerned with natural selection, and an adaptation to environments, and has focused primarily upon genes as 'replicators' and thus the blueprint for individual organisms.

In recent years there have been important developments in Darwinian medicine which is 'seeking evolutionary explanations for the susceptibility to disease' (Gerald and Higley, 2002) and also in areas such as socio-biology (see Wilson, 1975) and evolutionary psychology (see Barkow et al., 1992). However, Dawkins (2006) argues that the full significance of evolutionary theory in its impact on our understanding of all aspects of human development and functioning has yet to be realised. It is probably true to say that much of what is understood within the silos of academic and scientific research in respect of the evolutionary nature of life is not understood by the general public or they feel sceptical about such findings (see The

Academy of Medical Sciences, 2007). Much of this misunderstanding and scepticism, which is often reinforced by the popular media, concerns the nature of causality and the idea that there is a gene for this problem or for that behaviour, so if we can but identify the gene involved then we can solve the problem. Dawkins (2006: 3) makes the unequivocal statement that 'it is a fallacy … to suppose that genetically inherited traits are by definition fixed and unmodifiable'. He argues that, for example, we may be selfish but we can learn to be generous and altruistic, we may have a drive to biologically reproduce but we can still choose to use contraception. This development of conscious ways of acting that overcome our 'instinctive' ways of behaving is important in the development of not only culture in its broadest sense, but also an increasing capacity to overcome everyday challenges in our lives. Dawkins (2006) talks about the development of 'memes' which are cultural ideas such as religion or political causes which develop and grow in an evolutionary fashion, and it may be that when addressing issues such as addiction we then need to consider the search for recovery memes; in this respect it is interesting to note the development and growth of Twelve Step Fellowships around the world (see Chapter 3).

Hill and Newlin (2002) acknowledge that the application of evolutionary perspectives to human behaviours is not without its controversies and none more so than around ideas of genetic determinism. In fact as we shall see these controversies are implicit within an approach that has increasingly focused upon 'brain science' (see Robbins et al., 2007) and the idea of addiction as a brain disease. The risks are of viewing addiction as a fixed pathology that is impervious to change, and thus an area ripe for, at its extreme, a eugenicist approach, or at best reductions in the public funding of programmes of interventions. As we shall see simplistic accounts do not do justice to the complexity of these issues, or the rich vein of understanding that can emerge using some of these new paradigms.

For Nesse 'An evolutionary approach is wonderful because it poses fundamentally new questions' (2002: 470); but he also says that because these questions are new, they are hard to formulate clearly and even harder to answer. In the introduction to this book a number of key questions that are typically asked in the substance misuse field were outlined, which very much focus on differences between individuals in terms of drug use, misuse, addiction, and subsequent problems. This approach based upon individual differences is of course essentially pragmatic and diagnostic in nature so that people with problems or the potential for problems can be identified and dealt appropriately. However, the evolutionary perspective raises major questions about why all human beings are vulnerable to substance misuse and what is the ecological nature of the relationship between plants and animals within an evolutionary context (Nesse, 2002).

In response to the first question Nesse (2002) argues that drug use is what we should expect. This is because within the evolutionary environment our brains are shaped by natural selection and those brains regulate behaviour through chemical transmitters (see below). Given that the major drugs of misuse stimulate this system of chemical transmitters in a way that escalates drug taking then drug misuse becomes clearly inevitable. This then changes the focus onto questions of why substance misuse is not more widespread and why some people are able to control or stop their drug use. In addressing the second question Nesse (2002) states that plants over evolutionary time have developed strategies to protect themselves but also to ensure that they are propagated as well. Some chemicals such as caffeine, cocaine, and opiates are present in plants because they interact with the central nervous systems of animals to either kill them or make them feel ill. But plants also offer the attractions of flowers and pollen so that insects, for example, will feed off these and thus ensure pollination and reproduction.

An important question for Darwinian medicine is why natural selection has not eliminated vulnerability to certain diseases (Hill and Newlin, 2002); and furthermore when applying evolutionary theory to ideas around substance use and misuse a contradiction is faced in that evolutionary processes emphasise how behaviours benefit an organism, but in reality psychoactive substances have the capacity to cause a great deal of harm (Lende and Smith, 2002). One of the hypotheses given is that compromises in gene design may occur when genes that increase the risk of disease are able to confer benefits in other areas (Newlin and Hill, 2002) and also that adaptations develop to allow organisms to successfully reproduce within their environments (Lende and Smith, 2002). One of these adaptive processes is a phenomenon called hormesis (see Dudley, 2002) in which selective forces can evolve following a chronic but low level exposure to naturally occurring substances. The exposure follows a nutrient–toxin continuum where lower levels cause beneficial stimulation but higher levels cause stress and harm. Dudley (2002) argues that an evolutionary approach to hormesis assumes that natural selection maximises relative fitness and so organisms consequently develop metabolic systems to maximise the benefits and minimise the costs of exposure to low level concentrations of these naturally occurring substances.

It is proposed by Dudley (2000; 2002) that traditional approaches to addiction have focused upon the newness of psychoactive substances within the evolutionary context, with an historic exposure seen to be negligible. However, his central argument is that 'ethanol occupies a unique position in the nutritional ecology of *Homo sapiens*' (2000: 4) precisely because over at least 24 million years (and along with other animal fruit eaters), humans have regularly ingested naturally fermenting fruits. The argument that then follows is that, although not central to the various species of *Homo sapiens*, the consumption of fruit provided an important calorific intake, thus leading to the low level exposure to ethanol with corresponding physiological adaptations over the evolutionary time scale. Within this context 'alcoholism in modern humans may be viewed conceptually as a disease of nutritional excess' (Dudley, 2000: 7) in which genetically adapted behaviours forged over millennia become disadvantageous in an environment which gives easy access to nutritional substances such as ethanol.

Although the research in relation to alcohol suggests that there can be some health and social benefits associated with its consumption (see Edwards et al., 1995), increasingly evidence is suggesting that alcohol related harm is dose related where the risk of alcohol related harm increases exponentially for every unit drunk over and above the recommended levels indicating evidence for the hormesis hypothesis. In addition it does provide further evidence that supply and availability are key factors in determining the prevalence of alcohol related problems within a population.

In relation to drug use generally an important link between evolutionary theory and neurobiology is the role of the cortico-mesolimbic dopamine system (CMDA). The neurobiology of this is discussed below and the view that this is a hedonistic reward centre or pathway in the sense of chemical responses such as euphoria encouraging the use of psychoactive substances. However, Newlin (2002) utilises evolutionary theory to develop the self-perceived survival ability and reproductive fitness (SPFit) theory of substance use disorders. For Newlin the CMDA is not a reward centre as traditionally seen but is rather a survival and reproductive motivational system that has developed from the need for personal power and fitness in order to survive and reproduce. Within the evolutionary environment the need to survive and reproduce is of greater significance to animals than that of pleasure seeking and the CMDA responds to any environmental stimuli that is biologically relevant whereas a reward pathway would only respond to positive reinforcers that offer rewards. The application of this approach to our understanding of drug use is based upon the understanding that psychoactive substances inflate our feelings of power and sexual attractiveness.

Genomics

The genetic make up that we inherit from our parents has been shown to make an important contribution in increasing the risk of addictive behaviour, very often in interaction with wider environmental factors (Ball et al., 2007). A 'simplistic' summary of the foundations of genetics is given by Noble (2006) with the following:

- Genetic material is called DNA (deoxyribonucleic acid) which comes in long molecular strands made up of four chemicals called nucleotides, referred to by the letters A (Adenine), T (Thymine), C (Cytosine), and G (Guanine).
- A chromosome is a long DNA molecule, and some associated proteins, which is divided into sections called 'genes'.
- Each chromosome contains two complimentary strands of DNA wrapped around each other in a double helix, which makes a base pair.
- The human genome (which is the entire DNA of a human) is a sequence of three billion pairs of bases. Each one has been identified.
- Each of these bases provides a template to enable protein production, the sequence of which is encoded in the DNA. There is detailed knowledge of how this coding works and also of many of the proteins themselves that the DNA encodes.
- Chemicals are arranged in a specific way in each gene to produce specific proteins, of which there are about 100,000 that make up the human body. No protein is made unless it is coded for by a gene.
- Proteins form the backbone of all molecular interaction with the body, which allow cells to grow, divide, and form more cells.
- Every aspect of the body's function involves these proteins.

> What evidence might you look for to suggest a link between genetic make up and addiction?

Despite controversies and debates around our understanding of the human genome and its implications for treatments and broader interventions, the information that has been gathered from the mapping of the genome produces 'a single data set that encompasses the genetic basis of being human' and more than 1,400 human genes have been directly correlated with disease (Bentley, 2004: 440). In biology and in line with scientific method this reductionist approach seeks explanations for disease by breaking the phenomenon down into its component parts to see how these work. The above description of a genetic approach to the development of life gives rise to the danger of genetic determinism and simple cause and effect. Noble (2006) argues that the human genome is similar to a CD in that it carries digital information, but to say that the DNA code 'causes' life would be like saying that a CD 'caused' my experience of a particular piece of music. Similarly, in relation to drug use and addiction, we know that genes have an important part to play, but so do the particular drug (or drugs) being used and crucially the context in which they are used.

The observation has been made over a long period of time that there is a 'familial' nature to alcohol and drug abuse, which can often extend over generations of biologically related people. One of the main features of the evidence that stems from genetic research is that there is an increased statistical probability of the risk of developing a substance misuse problem, but this is not the same as establishing a direct causal relationship. The evidence for this increase in risk emanates from extended pedigree studies, studies of identical and fraternal twins, and studies of children who have been adopted away from their alcoholic parent(s). Hesselbrock and Hesselbrock (2006) state that although these studies cannot confirm the genetic hypothesis that there are genes that cause addiction, there is nonetheless persuasive evidence for genetic influences in increasing a vulnerability to addiction. It is important to realise that genetics are but one contribution to the biopsychsocial paradigm as some people have predisposing genes but do not manifest substance misuse problems and, likewise, some people develop problems who do not have predisposing genes. There is a lack of clarity around the role of genes and their influence upon addictive behaviour, with Nestler and Landsman (2001) arguing that based upon epidemiological studies it is estimated that 40–60% of an individual's risk for addiction, whether to alcohol, opiates, or cocaine is genetic; whereas Walters (2002, cited in Buckland, 2008) found a figure of between 24% and 36% based upon a meta analysis of 50 family, twin, and adoption studies, with the upper level based upon male only subjects with the most severe diagnosis. The point here is that the lower the heritability of the genes the lower the probability that this will have a significant effect.

Many of our illnesses and diseases are not simply due to our genetic inheritance, but emanate from agents in our surroundings (The Academy of Medical Science, 2007), and we have already stressed the importance of understanding drug use as an interaction between the individual, the drug, and the context in which it is used. There is plenty of evidence to suggest that environmental factors such as committed relationships moderate the 'expression' of predisposing genes (Hesselbrock and Hesselbrock, 2006).

This issue of gene expression is fundamental in understanding the nature of causality and also in overcoming the tendency towards genetic determinism with all its commensurate ethical and practical dangers. This determinism is based upon the understanding that genes are coded as sequences of DNA, which replicate themselves by being passed on to future generations; it is this process of replication which sees them described as causal agents. But the really important actors in developing life are the proteins and in comparison to which DNA is comparatively passive (Noble, 2006). It is the proteins that allow for gene expression, with the genes being the templates for the production of the specific protein. Although we are made up of genes inherited from our parents, at any time in our development certain genes can be either 'switched off' or 'switched on', and thus the proteins that they produce are either produced or not, with a part to play or not in the physiological process (Ball et al., 2007). Different environmental factors including exposure to psychoactive drugs all impact upon gene expression; and thus on the evidence summarised by Hesselbrock and Hesselbrock (2006) from twin studies demonstrating the importance of factors such as religious affiliation, marriage-like relationships, neighbourhood stability, and the local availability of alcohol.

Addiction as a 'brain disease'

One of the criticisms of the classical disease model posited by Heather and Robertson (1997, see Chapter 3) was that it was not clearly formulated, in the sense that there were logically a number of differing models based upon notions of physiology, psychopathology, and acquired disease. However, in recent times the idea of addiction as a disease of the brain has gained rapid acceptance, particularly in the USA. Whilst this has been aided by the advances in the scientific areas highlighted, it is probably true to say that this has raised as many questions as have been answered, with a primary focus still on the ethics of policy and interventions and with particular reference to coerced interventions within the criminal justice system.

The idea of a 'brain disease' as a social problem is, for example, clearly argued by Dackis and O'Brien (2005: 1431) who state that scientific evidence supports 'a disease concept of addiction based on neuronal mechanisms, heritability, treatment responses and characteristic progressive clinical course'. They make the same arguments about helping people who are the victims of disease as the Temperance Movement did for people with alcohol problems in the late nineteenth and early twentieth centuries. For Dackis and O'Brien, it is precisely the lack of a humane disease perspective that allows society to discriminate and criminalise people who are afflicted by these problems. It has been suggested that what the developments in brain science allow for is an appeal to traditional disease perspectives but with the added legitimacy and authority of modern science (Hall et al., 2003).

The neurobiological process sees addiction as a cycle, starting with the light side in which drug seeking behaviour and drug use emanate from a failure to suppress impulses; drug use leads to euphoric experiences which positively reinforce (a positive reinforcer is an event that increases the probability of a response on which it is contingent) the activity through activated reward pathways; neuroadaptations in the form of withdrawal and tolerance occur which leads to the dysregulation of the reward system; withdrawal and increased tolerance then lead into the dark side where drug craving and negative reinforcement (a negative reinforcer is an activity that when stopped increases the probability of the response on which it is contingent) occur which in turn leads to a loss of control and poor decision making; and as a consequence of which there is an increased likelihood of drug seeking and drug using behaviour (Dackis and O'Brien, 2005).

Leshner (2007) argues that addiction along with other brain diseases such as stroke, Alzheimers, and schizophrenia are not purely biological in nature, but that there are social aspects as well. However an important difference is that addiction usually begins with the voluntary use of a drug and we need to consider why people would use substances that are likely to be damaging. We have already seen that evolutionary theory provides us with some useful insights into this, but one of the key areas of research is to understand the changes that occur in the brain in the transition from normal to addictive behaviour (Volkow and Fowler, 2000) and what causes 'an addicted person to lose control of drug-taking behaviour even when experiencing serious drug related harm?' (Hyman and Malenka, 2001: 695).

Within the brain disease model the essential components of the Classical Disease Model and of Dependence Syndromes remain, namely tolerance, dependence and withdrawal, and a loss of control. Tolerance is defined as the need for an increased dose to maintain a stable effect and this increased usage in turn can exacerbate molecular changes that lead to addiction. It is argued by Hyman and Malenka (2001) that, despite the conflation of the terms 'dependence' and 'addiction', in a scientific sense these are not the same. Dependence is to be seen as adaptations that occur in cells, circuits, or organ systems in response to the stimulation caused by excessive drug use. Whilst both psychological and physical withdrawal symptoms occur when the drug use ceases, these do not necessarily lead to compulsive use. It is this compulsion which is at the heart of 'addiction' and where the cravings for a drug are no longer based upon pleasure, but the need for it. Koob suggests that drug addiction should be seen as 'a disorder that progresses from impulsivity to compulsivity' (2006: 25). This is also conceptualised as a shift from the 'light' side to the 'dark' side of drug taking.

The study of physiology has identified that differing physiological processes have a common purpose, namely to create a dynamic stability for an organism in the face of stress (Buchman, 2002). The dynamic nature of organisms is important here and follows from their evolutionary drive to survive, allowing for organisms to act to restore and compensate for any challenges to that survival that may occur. The process of maintaining physiological stability is called homeostasis. This is described by Koob and Le Moal as holding 'all the parameters of the organisms' internal milieu within limits that allow an organism to survive' (2001: 101). Stability is maintained by the component systems of the organism working together to respond to an acute challenge and to maintain the 'set points' that the system requires for working effectively within its homeostatic parameters. Homeostasis is thus described as 'a self regulating process for maintaining body parameters around a set point critical for survival' (McEwen, 2000, cited in Koob and Le Moal, 2001: 101). In contrast to homeostasis the principle of allostasis occurs when an organism is put under such chronic pressure that it has to maintain the stability of the organism outside of the normal homeostatic range, by resetting the parameters of the system at a new set point. This is an adaptive and dynamic process that maintains stability through change (Koob and Le Moal, 2001).

In respect of drug use and addiction the allostatic perspective is seen 'as the process of maintaining apparent reward function stability through changes in brain reward and stress mechanisms' (Koob, 2006: 41). Within this context the initial light sided hedonic effects are experienced but these give way to the darker side of withdrawal when drug use is terminated. This is a process of counter-adaptation in which the dark side increases with repeated exposure and is slow to decay (Koob, 2006).

Not all of the major drugs of misuse cause physical dependency (defined as adaptations in the brain from drug use that lead to directly observable changes in bodily functions), for example alcohol and opiates do, but cocaine does not. It has often been argued that avoidance of the discomfort of withdrawal symptoms explains compulsive use. However, Hyman and Malenka (2001) point out that if this were the case then after a few weeks of careful management when the withdrawal symptoms disappear there should no longer be a problem. Yet people can relapse long after the withdrawal symptoms are gone and, for drugs which do not cause physical dependence, when the physical symptoms are absent and the emotional symptoms variable. It is therefore argued that in themselves the issues of tolerance, dependence, and withdrawal are not sufficient to explain compulsive drug taking or a relapse after a prolonged period of time (Hyman and Malenka, 2001).

The brain disease model conceptualises the disease as one that is caused by the adaptive changes that occur in the reward centres of the brain which have developed within an evolutionary context to ensure the survival of the organism and its species (Dackis and O'Brian, 2005). These areas of the brain have developed to regulate and reinforce our behaviour towards meeting the basic human needs of food, drink, sex, and social interaction (Bickell and Potenza, 2006). These areas of the brain which are implicated in drug taking behaviour have been termed as the 'mesolimbic reward system' which comprises the ventral tegmental area and the basal forebrain. Communication within the brain is dependent upon the release of neuro-transmitters and within this neural circuitry circuits for the reinforcing effects of drugs have evolved along with four main neurotransmitter systems (Koob, 2006). These are the mesolimbic dopamine system, the opioid peptide system, the gamma-aminobutyric acid system, and the endocannibinoid system. When experiencing a withdrawal from psychoactive drugs dysphoria, anxiety, and panic attacks occur, and there is also an increase in the body's chemicals that produce a stress reaction and thus lead to drug seeking behaviour (Koob, 2006). (For a full introductory discussion of these issues see Koob, 2006.)

> Go back to Chapter 5 and make the links between psychological learning processes and neuro processes.

Relevance for interventions

Ball et al. (2007) argue that although the UK government amongst others has raised the issue of genetic profiling at birth as an important component of health management, at best this can only have a limited role in preventing substance misuse. This approach is limited precisely because gene expression is so contingent on other social and psychological factors that it becomes almost impossible to predict (see also Buckland, 2008). The question of whether insights from evolutionary biology are of any relevance to clinicians is raised by Chick (2002) who asks whether these simply allow us to apportion less blame to individuals who harm themselves through the use of psychoactive substances.

The Academy of Medical Sciences (2008) suggests that to date these new insights have had little impact upon the development of new medicines to treat addiction, although the field is rich with promise with substantial investment. Most of the focus to date has been on pharmacological interventions to maintain abstinence. The difficulty here, as highlighted by Goldstein (2001) and Hall (2006), is that as with all medical regimes compliance is a problem, which can often lead to calls for coerced treatments.

The brain disease model seen within the context of genetic and evolutionary theory is complex, but is also an important building block towards viewing addiction as an example of a complex adaptive system which will be discussed in Chapter 8. As we saw in Chapter 3, at the heart of the discussions about 'disease' are notions of personal responsibility and the degree to which individuals can be held responsible for their actions. Advances in our understanding of human behaviour clearly demonstrate that the origins of this behaviour are complex and involve profound biological processes that are also adaptational in nature, involving an interaction between genes and environment. We can therefore conclude that, although we have a very good understanding of the biological nature of addiction and the changes that occur, medically this has not taken us much further forward. Pharmacology has a vitally important role to play, whether through substitute prescribing, managing withdrawal symptoms, or reducing craving for substances, but only as an adjunct to wider psychological and social approaches.

Conclusion

In the next chapter we will discuss the evidence for effective interventions and especially psychosocial approaches with particular reference to motivational approaches. A key part of effective working for clinicians and practitioners is the need to develop empathic relationships, and talking therapies which can overcome even those problems that have a biological basis such as mental health problems and addiction. One of the limitations arising from much biological research in this area is that it has been carried out on animals which has generated a great deal of new knowledge, although as Chick (2002) argues this needs to be tested carefully to avoid rapid and potentially dangerous applications to humans. In addition to this is the capacity for human animals to act in ways that are not driven by instinct or 'genetic programming' and as we shall see in Chapter 8 complex systems tend towards higher rather than lower order solutions to problems. These higher order solutions need to be based upon the idea that personal responsibility is an aspiration that all of us work towards, but is not something we are born with. Much of the focus has been on identifying of the genes of addiction (in a reductionist sense) whereas the focus should perhaps be on higher order 'recovery memes'. This of course fits with some of the psychological perspectives outlined in Chapter 5 and partly explains both the success and appeal of talking therapies, whether Twelve Step in nature or part of the various cognitive and behavioural approaches. It is also clear that environmental factors in the form of family and peer group are crucial in determining how we are socialised into 'being responsible', as well as our exposure to psychoactive substances. Over the course of time, due to the way our cortico-mesolimbic dopamine systems have evolved, all of us will struggle with impulsive behaviour which can become problematic for some people; if there is a genetic component then it is only a part of the overall picture. This appreciation of our common humanity, which is clearly demonstrated by cutting edge research in neurobiology, then needs to form the basis for our interventions. When Heather and Robertson (1997) critiqued the classical disease perspective for lacking coherence and not being clear about whether the disease was pathological, psychopathological, or acquired in nature, possibly they could not have imagined that potentially all three elements could be involved!

Useful resources

Dawkins, R. (2006) *The Selfish Gene* (30th anniversary edition). Oxford: Oxford University Press.

Noble, D. (2006) *The Music of Life: Biology Beyond Genes*. Oxford: Oxford University Press.

The Human Genome Project – www.ornl.gov/sci/techresources/Human_Genome/home.shtml

7

Interventions and Equivocal Outcomes

The aims of this chapter are to:

- discuss the 'equivalence paradox' in relation to outcomes from treatments that include Twelve Step facilitation, cognitive behavioural and motivational approaches
- discuss the importance of empathy and motivational working
- highlight the case management context of service provision
- highlight the importance of working with relapse
- lay the foundations for the final chapters.

In each of the preceding chapters we have considered some of the ways in which theories and models of addiction relate to appropriate interventions, to prevent or ameliorate problems associated with the use of psychoactive substances. It is quite clear from reviewing the development of interventions over the course of the last 150 years or so, that at times theory and practice have had significant impacts upon policy and the subsequent commissioning of services. The obvious example of this is the way that the classical disease model developing out of the Temperance Movement allowed for the development of specialist services for 'alcoholics'. However, over the course of time our understanding of drug use and specifically the idea of 'addiction' has developed in response to research findings (particularly alcoholics returning to controlled drinking), which has matched practitioner experiences (hence the development of the idea of a Dependence Syndrome), and the importance of psychological talking therapies to train addicts in what are essentially coping skills for dealing with the risk and reality of relapse. As often occurs, new research promises new interventions which are then picked up by policy makers and commissioners. But the key questions within this is 'does treatment work?' by what standard or measure should this be judged, and are some treatments better than others?

> Is treatment an appropriate term to cover all aspects of interventions with people using and misusing substances?

In thinking about the nature of interventions and services to address drug use, and its associated problems, it will be argued that these interventions and the settings in which they occur are examples of complex systems in which theory, policy, clinical, and helping skills meet in either formal or informal settings. The idea of complex systems will be discussed in detail in Chapter 8, but the purpose of this chapter is to build up to this by reviewing what is known from the extensive literature on effective interventions within the field of substance misuse and to discuss the implications for practitioners and people experiencing problematic drug use. The aims of this chapter are then to review the evidence for what is effective in addressing substance misuse and on the basis of this to lay the groundwork for a discussion in the final chapter on developing more responsive systems of intervention. The idea of an ethical approach based upon our scientific knowledge as being central to working effectively in the overcoming of problems with addiction will be advocated. There is nothing new here of course as the research consistently demonstrates the importance of the working relationship between service user and service provider, in ways which express an open, warm, empathic, and motivational approach to the person and the problems involved (see Miller and Rollnick, 2002; Miller, 2006). But through the lens of complexity we can add to the argument in shaping interventions which are less judgemental and coercive and reflect our common experiences with psychoactive substances of one kind or another; the logic of the biopsychosocial paradigm and its evolutionary context is that we are all susceptible to an addiction to substances as well as other behaviours and are likely to experience problems associated with that use.

What is the evidence base for interventions?

In the literature it is recognised that any approach to addressing problematic drug use has to acknowledge the range of ways in which people change their behaviour, from self-help through to intensive residential and inpatient settings (see DiClemente and Prochaska, 1998; and Orford, 2008). As we have seen these interventions arise from bio-medical, psychological, and social approaches, incorporating a whole range of these from policy approaches to control the supply and availability of particular substances, through to health and social policy designed to address the effects of use, through to harm reduction interventions, Twelve Step (and other self-help approaches) and psychological talking therapies. In Chapter 2 it was argued that governments across the industrialised world have searched for answers to health and social problems, based upon interventions that have demonstrable 'evidence based' outcomes.

> What do you think constitutes a good outcome from treatment and why? How should those outcomes be evidenced?

The scientific basis of medicine has traditionally sought to find evidence to understand the aetiology of a disorder and to provide the correct treatment approach with the appropriate dosage for the severity of the problem. However, as Humphreys and Tucker (2002) point out, alcohol and drug misuse is not the same as an acute medical problem for which short term medical interventions can provide lasting improvements without having to significantly change the patient's environment or behaviour. One of the central features of addiction as a chronic relapsing condition then becomes critical to this discussion and the extent to which individuals are held responsible for their actions and are able to access treatments despite successive relapses. This has particularly been an issue in an era of central government seeking to reduce health and welfare costs through the rationing and targeting of scarce resources via the development of 'internal markets' in the provision of health and social care, with the advent of 'care management' and the role of the Care Manager.

In the fields of health and social welfare the idea of 'Evidence-based Policy', has become central to the thinking of politicians, commissioners of services, and practitioners. This approach, which Pawson (2006: 1) refers to as 'a new millennium big idea', was very much at the centre of New Labour's thinking on social policy when coming to power in 1997 and in the treatment sector, particularly in relation to criminal justice, is referred to as 'What Works' (see McGuire, 1995). In 1997 New Labour had ambitious plans for modernising the British economy as well as the National Health Service and the range of social and welfare services provided by or through government funding. For New Labour and the European Commission this meant 'scientific and other experts play[ing] an increasingly significant role in preparing and monitoring decisions … The Institutions rely on specialist expertise to anticipate and identify the nature of the problems' (European Union, 2001, cited in Pawson, 2006: 2). The importance of this is that there has been an important and growing relationship between the sciences and the development of policies that affect our everyday lives, and this is just as true when dealing with substance misuse as it is when modelling the economy or addressing heart disease.

In the 1970s the establishment of the concept of the Dependence Syndrome had opened up the possibility for new treatment modalities based upon a thorough assessment of the clinical needs of the individual person. It is important to remember that this was occurring within a rather pessimistic view of rehabilitation generally in dealing with a range of problematic behaviours. In the early 1970s, a criminologist called Robert Martinson (1974) had reviewed therapeutic programmes in American prisons and came to some conclusions about their effectiveness. The misrepresentation of his findings was to have a profound effect upon the nature of therapeutic programmes across the developed world and ultimately led to his suicide. Although he did observe that the programmes appeared to be having very little overall effect to justify their existence, he came to this conclusion with the following caveats concerning methodology: firstly, he thought that some of the programmes may have been having beneficial results, but that the research methods of the time may not have been sophisticated enough to detect them; secondly, that the principles the programmes were based upon may have been sound, but that the delivery was not good enough; or thirdly, that the theoretical basis of the programmes may have been flawed insofar as they treated a diverse and social phenomenon like offending behaviour in a medicalised and unitary way. Despite the questions that Martinson raised, the impact of this piece of research was far reaching and led to the perception that 'nothing works' in addressing issues such as offending behaviour and substance misuse problems. This led to a period of disinvestment in programmes of rehabilitation, with more of an onus on incarcerating people for their crimes particularly with a 'War on Drugs' approach to substance misuse.

In 1990 the Institute of Medicine (IOM) produced a seminal document entitled *Broadening the Base for the Treatment of Alcohol Problems* in which it specifically addressed the question of 'does treatment work?' In response to this the IOM argued that it was too simplistic a question, with the additional hazard of evoking too simplistic responses; therefore the IOM argued that given the complex nature of both the question and its potential answers that the question should be reframed. The IOM argued for a reframing of the question on the basis of the inappropriate implication that there is a unitary phenomenon (the assumption of the classical disease approach) to be dealt with rather than the reality of alcohol problems existing in multiplicity and diversity. In relation to this it was argued that the question also overlooks the range of therapeutic interventions that actually exist, in contrast to there being one standardised approach. Additionally the focus of the question is on the effectiveness of one single episode of treatment, whereas again the reality is that for many people more than one period of treatment might be necessary, and often of different kinds. The IOM went on to argue that within the question there is too much focus on treatment at the expense of other factors that might contribute to outcomes from an intervention, namely the characteristics of the individual seeking treatment, the nature of the problem itself, and also the post treatment context, for example will a homeless drinker still be homeless after treatment? Finally the IOM questioned whether it is possible to have an absolute standard for outcome that the question implies. In this sense should we be considering hard and fast measures of abstinence or consumption reduction or might we consider improvements in housing or relationships as important goals in their own right for treatment services (see Fiorentine, 1998)? In an era of managed care, this becomes an important question for Care Managers who are purchasing packages of care for service users with a multiplicity of needs, and who are also performance managed and required to justify the funding of their services through demonstrating outcome measurements.

Despite the accumulating evidence of the importance of motivational approaches (Raistrick et al., 2006), within the context of the UK, one of the striking features of the last ten years or so has been the increased use of 'coerced treatments' within the criminal justice system. The rapid expansion of criminal justice interventions has fundamentally impacted upon the delivery of services (see Seddon et al., 2008), with a range of health and social care professionals and organisations working in partnership with the agencies of law and order. The literature on criminal justice coerced interventions supports another aspect of the equivalence paradox by suggesting that these interventions are no better nor worse than voluntaristic ones (see McSweeney et al., 2006). However, we need to be clear about our terms of reference; it is argued that the differences between coerced and voluntary approaches are not necessarily dichotomous in nature but represent more of a spectrum of 'motivations' to address problematic behaviour. Despite this it is quite clear that the consequences of being coerced either by pressure from friends or family are very different to pressure applied by the state and the apparatus of the criminal justice system. As an addict I may lose my friends and family, but this is not going to deprive me of my liberty, or lose me my job, or put me in prison. This is an important issue because within the debate about the equivalence paradox, some commentators argue that we know that coercion and punishment are not effective strategies for dealing with addiction (see Miller and Rollnick, 2002; Miller, 2006). This will form an important part of the argument in the next chapter.

Assumptions regarding interventions

According to Lindstrom (1992: 40) we can identify three major questions which are central to debates concerning treatments for alcohol problems (and thus drug problems and psychotherapeutic approaches in general). Firstly, is treatment effective? Secondly, do therapies vary in efficacy, and thirdly, is there a superior therapy? Lindstrom argues that the assumptions about treatment research into alcohol dependency can be classified into four major categories based upon their response to these questions, as can be seen in Table 7.1.

TABLE 7.1   *Assumptions regarding the treatment of alcohol problems*

	Is treatment effective?	Do therapies vary in efficacy?	Is there a superior therapy?
The technique hypothesis	Yes	Yes	Yes
The matching hypothesis	Yes	Yes	No
The non-specific hypothesis	Yes	No	–
The natural healing hypothesis	No	–	–

Source: taken from Lindstrom, 1992, by permission of Oxford University Press.

The 'technique hypothesis' expects to find an approach or setting that is superior for all patients with a given diagnosis and thus drives the search for the most effective treatment based upon robust scientific principles. This has informed, for example, the psychoanalytic school of thought from the work of Freud and his disciples through to the cognitive-behavioural approaches of the 'What Works' agenda of the National Probation Service (see below). The 'matching hypothesis' recognises interaction effects between the patient and other treatment variables such as programme content and delivery style. This approach seeks to match patient characteristics with treatment approaches, rather than finding a single programme that is effective for all. The 'non-specific hypothesis' recognises that treatment can be effective, but that because all treatments produce beneficial and equivalent results it does not matter which approach is used. The benefits stem from processes that are common to the range of interventions and so it is important to identify those processes for the enhancement of existing therapies. At the other end of the spectrum from the 'technique hypothesis' is that of 'natural healing', which argues that the outcomes from interventions are no better than for those that are experienced as a result of spontaneous remission or influences beyond the control of the therapist. Whilst there is plenty of evidence to suggest that the majority of people with substance misuse problems resolve their difficulties without recourse to formal treatment (see Orford, 2002, Chapter 13, 'The Place of Expert Help'), clearly there are people who do not. As has been argued throughout this book, these people can experience intense suffering, and be the cause of suffering to others, which therefore means that there is a practical and ethical obligation to try and alleviate that suffering. The ways in which interventions have been constructed and delivered are a matter of controversy, as can be seen from Lindstrom's questions and the treatment typologies arising from them.

Asking the right questions

With these concerns in mind the IOM (1990: 143) suggests an expansion of the original question to include the following: 'Which kinds of individuals, with what kinds of alcohol problems, are likely to respond to what kinds of treatments by achieving what kinds of goals when delivered by what kinds of practitioners?' The IOM called for more emphasis on which interventions worked for which people and in which circumstances. It is argued that, 'No single treatment approach is effective for all persons with alcohol problems. A more promising strategy involves assigning patients to alternative treatments based on specific needs and characteristics of patients' (see Project MATCH, 2005). Since then two major studies, Project MATCH in the USA and the UK Alcohol Treatment Trial (UKATT), have taken place. Project MATCH took a cohort of 1,726 problem drinkers and allocated people to either Cognitive Behavioural Therapy Coping Skills (CBT), Twelve Step Facilitation (TSF), or Motivational Enhancement Therapy (MET) (Project MATCH Research Group, 1997). For the UKATT trial a total of 720 people were randomised to MET or Social Behaviour and Network Therapy (SBNT). It is not my intention to outline these approaches in detail but suffice it to say that TSF is based upon the tenets of Alcoholics Anonymous; CBT is a standard psychological approach; MET has been developed from Motivational Interviewing; and SBNT contains elements aimed at developing positive social support for change from the community reinforcement approach, marital therapy, network therapy, relapse prevention, and social skills training (UKATT

Research Group, 2001). Both of these studies have failed to find any significant differences in outcomes from the treatments compared despite very different underlying theories of service delivery.

The outcome equivalence paradox

At the heart of this discussion is the so called 'outcome equivalence paradox' which argues that despite a whole range of interventions being available, and delivered from apparently contrasting theoretical bases, the outcomes are broadly the same for all treatments (Orford, 2008). Likewise in a study by Imel and Wampold (2008), who meta-analysed studies which directly compared two 'bona fide' psychological treatments, they argue that their results are consistent with an emphasis on therapeutic processes common across different treatments (such as the relationship between therapist and client) and common mechanisms of change, rather than specific techniques supposedly stimulating specific mechanisms linked to a specific complaint. This supports the argument that the search for more effective therapeutic programmes is wrong because it is not the specific programme which matters but 'common factors' which cut across these programmes, such as entering a therapeutic setting within which the patient expects to be helped to get better. The credibility of the therapy to both patient and therapist is essential, as is its ability to make ordered sense of the patient's 'disorder' and in so doing to structure a route out of that disorder which generates optimism. This needs to provide a platform for engaging the client in their recovery and for the therapist to have the ability to create a supportive environment which facilitates these processes. Perhaps the greatest common factor lies in the service users, who will have reached a point where they desperately want to get better, will have realised they need help to do so, and will have sought formal treatment.

The evidence from these studies and supported by the evidence from MATCH and UKATT argues that the outcomes differed little, overall, between therapies and that there were few indications that certain types of patient benefited more from one therapy than another. The findings from both MATCH and UKATT suggest the importance of a common factor model with a focus on the core processes of change common to all successful interventions. The idea of core processes of change was central to the trans-theoretical model of intentional behavioural change as discussed in Chapter 5 and drew upon a range of cognitive, behavioural, humanist, and existential therapies.

The implications for service provision

So what are the implications of this equivalence paradox for people suffering with addiction, for policy makers, commissioners, and practitioners, or in the words of Pawson (2006: 1) exactly 'how does "evidence" speak to "power"', and 'what hope is there for nuptials between "knowing and doing?"' Orford (2008) argues that the time has now come to accept that in most respects all of these interventions are doing exactly the same thing, but that certain forms of intervention have received more attention than others, thus reflecting researcher bias and the appearance of more research evidence for those specific treatments. He also suggests that this is a continued belief in the technique hypothesis and the illusion that it is only a matter of time before we find the best treatment or ways to match people to the most appropriate treatment.

Navigating the system

In line with its commitment to an evidence based approach and with the establishment of the National Treatment Agency in 2001, the New Labour government in the UK for the first time took a nationally coordinated approach to dealing with treatment for illicit drug use. At the strategic level the NTA works through local Drug Action Teams to address local priorities, but within the Models of Care Framework (MOC). This framework outlines the range of services that is to be commissioned nationally for adult substance misusers and is to be available in every part of England. In line with other national service frameworks (see Chapter 2) the aim of this approach is to ensure equity, parity, and consistency in the commissioning and provision of services.

The National Treatment Agency (www.nta.nhs.uk) provides information about the types of treatment available for substance misuse problems and defines treatment as 'a range of interventions that are intended to remedy an identified drug-related problem or condition relating to a person's physical, psychological or social (including legal) wellbeing. Structured drug treatment follows assessment and is delivered according to a care plan, with clear goals, which is regularly reviewed with the client'. In the previous chapters we have discussed some of these interventions and alluded to others, but the list of interventions that the NTA gives is:

- advice and information
- harm reduction
- community prescribing

- counselling and psychological support (including cognitive-behavioural approaches, coping skills, relapse prevention, motivational working, and family therapy)
- structured day programmes
- detoxification
- rehabilitation
- aftercare.

Importantly the 'MOC advocates a whole system approach to meeting the multiple needs of drug and alcohol misusers' (National Treatment Agency, 2004: 9; 2006) by recognising the range of drug related harms and thus also the range of differing agencies involved in drug related work. The MOC framework is split into four tiers:

1 Tier One consists of a range of drug related interventions that can be provided by generic services such as housing and social services, very often in conjunction with specialist substance misuse services. For example, tenancy support or debt counselling are important support mechanisms for some drug users.
2 Tier Two is concerned with interventions that engage people in drug treatment, providing support prior to structured treatment, and helping to retain people within the treatment system. This may also involve harm reduction interventions (see Chapter 4) and services for those people who do not need or want structured interventions.
3 Tier Three includes all substitute prescribing interventions, as well as structured care planned community based services following a comprehensive assessment.
4 Tier Four interventions include the provision of specialised residential drug treatment which is care planned and care coordinated.

As well as providing treatment tiers defined by different levels of intensity and structure the framework identifies the importance of screening, assessment and referral, the need for care coordination, and the establishment of integrated care pathways. But what the MOC does not stipulate in relation to structured community and residential care is what the nature of those programmes should be. Although all organisations receiving funding from the state to provide substance misuse services have to comply with organisational standards, as well as occupational standards for their staff, these can be medical, psychological, or Twelve Step programmes. The MOC argues that there has 'been a somewhat limited consensus among clinicians, other providers and commissioners about the essential components of specialist substance misuse treatment services and limited recognition of links with other health and social care support services' (National Treatment Agency, 2001: 6). In navigating this 'whole system' to establish integrated care pathways and to access resources the Care Manager has a crucial role to play.

The development of care management processes and the role of the Care Manager has fundamentally changed the ways in which individuals are provided for in receiving state funded interventions for a whole range of social and medical needs. This approach has been developed across the industrialised world, partly in response to rising health and welfare bills for central government and partly because of the growing complexity of the problems that professionals are working with (see McKay and McLellan, 1998). There are, however, differing models of care/case management with little research evidence about the ways in which they are implemented or their relative effectiveness (McSweeney and Hough, 2006). The initial UK approach was enshrined in the NHS and Community Care Act (1990), which had six main objectives (Means et al., 2003):

1   To ensure that available resources (including welfare benefits) are used in the most effective way to meet individual needs.
2   to restore and maintain independence by enabling people to live in the community wherever possible.
3   to work to prevent disability and illness in people of all ages.
4   to treat service users with respect and to provide equal opportunities for all.
5   to utilise existing strengths and resources to promote individual choice and self-determination.
6   to promote partnerships between service users, carers and service providers in all sectors (statutory, not for profit and private).

> What do you see as the strengths and weaknesses of care/case management approaches?

It was envisaged that this approach would be implemented through a comprehensive assessment of the service user's situation and also their carers if necessary; a negotiation of the care package between service user, carers, and the relevant agencies which could meet those identified needs within the resources available; the implementation, monitoring, and review of that package to consider outcomes and any changes to service provision that may be required (Means et al., 2003). This model is designed to maximise the resources available from all sectors, and also to promote service user choice, and has been developed in social work practice, mental health and offender management, though is not without controversy. However, it is the extant model within the UK context in the way that the NTA via the DATs works in partnership with health and social services and it raises some important issues about effective working practice in addressing substance misuse problems.

The reality of people presenting to services with a range of needs (including poly drug and alcohol problems, health and mental health problems, criminal involvement, unemployment, housing issues, and relationship difficulties) is that the service user has to access a range of different agencies (see Chapter 1 for the range of problems that people present to services with).

While this will be supported and monitored by a Care Manager, from a practice or clinical point of view, that Care Manager may not be directly involved in all aspects of the delivery of services as other specialist agencies will be providing for these needs, which can lead to an experience which is fragmented and confusing for the service user. This important issue was picked up by Partridge (2004) who conducted research for the Home Office. Partridge found that offenders valued the continuity and consistency in seeing the same person each time to talk to and share their problems with, as opposed to more people being involved in their supervision.

Working with relapse

The role of the Care/Case Manager is vital not only in assessing for and brokering packages of care, but also in helping the service user to navigate their way through 'the system' (McSweeney and Hough, 2006). In this respect the Care Manager has an essential role to play, in line with the research evidence to support recovery through:

- comprehensively assessing needs
- building a motivational relationship
- ensuring an appropriate extensity and sequencing of service provision
- retaining people in services through effectively supporting relapse prevention and relapse management strategies.

Fundamental to this approach is a more realistic evaluation of outcome based upon a chronic care perspective. This idea is developed by McLellan (2002) who argues that reviews of the literature demonstrate very similar treatment adherence and treatment relapse rates between addictions and diseases such as diabetes, hypertension, and asthma. McLellan provides evidence to show that when people are prescribed medications for these chronic illnesses less than 50% continued to take them as prescribed, less than 30% complied with required behavioural changes such as weight loss, dietary restrictions or exercise regimes, and that between 40–60% relapsed every year. On the basis of our understanding of the biopsychosocial paradigm of addiction, the question that is asked is whether a chronic care perspective helps us to develop more suitable and responsive services. In particular this begs the question of how we should view relapse, and what the implications should be of relapse not only for the individual concerned but also for the services that they have been utilising. Within this discussion it is important to remember that not all people who use substances are chronically addicted, and can recover without any formal treatment, but some are and will experience multiple relapses and a range of related harms (McLellan, 2002).

Should relapse be viewed in a positive or a negative way?

Given that relapse is one of the accepted defining features of addiction, it is not an issue that should cause surprise and is something to be expected, in the same way that is so with other chronic conditions. However, there is a tendency for relapse to be seen as a failure, of the individual 'going back to square one', and this is usually a reason for people not being allowed to continue with the services they were receiving. Relapse is not then a sign of poor motivation, and can be extremely distressing for the individual concerned, but neither does it indicate a failure of treatment or that there is not hope a of recovery. Of particular importance is the fact that a person does not need to hit 'rock bottom' before they can get further help (Ranganathan, 2005). It also has to be acknowledged that relapse is a risky business and in the extreme can lead to death, or other serious incidents, and therefore it becomes important to try and maintain a working relationship with the individual so that the gains already made in treatment are not lost. We know from the research literature that maintaining contact with services and the length of time in treatment are important indicators of a good outcome. It has been suggested by the NTORS research that a minimum of 90 days is essential for beneficial effects and also that episodes of treatment can have cumulative effects (this fits with the approach of the TTM). All of these become important reasons to keep people within services rather than forcing them to leave due to a relapse, which means that we need effective strategies of relapse management and continuing care. Unfortunately, within the UK context there is anecdotal evidence to suggest that the funders of services are limiting periods of treatment (particularly in more expensive residential settings) to 90 days, rather than seeing this as a minimum.

Learning from self-help groups

In responding to drug and alcohol problems the self-help organisations, and the ways in which they operate, have much to teach the professional sectors. Organisations such as AA and NA operate 24/7 and 365 days a year, and in most areas of the developed world there will be a fellowship meeting in most towns and cities (see Humphreys, 2004). In contrast most professional agencies will have set opening hours and be closed evenings, weekends, and Bank Holidays. Some of the lessons to be drawn from self-help approaches are discussed by Humphreys and Tucker (2002) in relation to creating more flexible and responsive service provision. They argue that interventions should be made on demand, ideally the same day that help is requested, as attendance drops rapidly with increased waiting times, whereas rapid treatment entry does not seem to correlate with subsequent treatment dropout. This is an interesting point because traditionally one of the reasons for refusing access to services has been as a result of poor motivation or being motivated for the wrong reasons. A cursory look at some materials from residential rehabs will often show the reasons for why some people will not be accepted, which may include issues such as having an outstanding court case or concurrent mental health problems. The evidence covered in Chapter 1 clearly demonstrates that these issues come with the territory and furthermore there is evidence to suggest (see Fiorentine, 1998) that getting people into services is important precisely to build the motivation for change. At the very least if addiction is to be seen as an impairment of the motivational system (West, 2006) then ambivalence is to be expected in the early stages of seeking help, which can appear as chaotic behaviour, by saying one thing and doing another. Humphreys and Tucker (2002) go on to suggest that, in the early stages of treatment, a harm reduction approach is more appropriate than the requirement for complete abstinence, as the latter may deter some people from seeking help. This client centred approach is obviously in keeping with a working relationship that seeks to build motivation rather than impose it.

> How can your agency or an agency that you know become more responsive to the needs of its service users?

Being an Agent of Hope

Finally, and perhaps most importantly, we know from the general psychotherapy literature (see Yalom, 2005) that one of key ingredients that effective helping has to offer is 'hope', and so any organisation or worker who wants to be effective has to be an 'Agent or Agency of Hope'. In practice this means building motivation that is directed towards the service user's levels and sources of motivation to change and working on successes rather than accentuating the negative. It is this that provides the reasons for change; that by reducing or stopping drug use real improvements in quality of life can occur, namely that an intervention or a series of interventions offers is something that is qualitatively different to what the person is currently experiencing. Westerberg (1998) argues that in this area of work we do not talk much about success but tend to focus on failure in the form of relapse. Once again this focus on failure revolves around black and white, all or nothing thinking, around a fixed point of you have either succeeded or you have not. It is clear that recovery from addiction is a process, and sometimes a lengthy one, that involves relapse, which at its best can provide a learning opportunity to try and do things differently. For Westerberg (1998: 305) 'success predicts success', with success defined as 'just one point on a continuum of outcomes that might be thought of as going from no change in any behaviour as a result of therapeutic intervention to the living of a full and productive life'.

> In what ways are you able to develop your role as an Agent of Hope for people with substance misuse problems?

To achieve the possibility of change it is important that the full range of interventions is available, from harm reduction through to psychological interventions to build self-efficacy and self-esteem, and to address dual diagnosis issues through to social supports such as housing and employment schemes. This is a complicated world even for the professionals engaged in it, so how much more confusing can it be for anxious and vulnerable service users? The role of the Care/Case Manager then becomes a critical one.

Conclusion

In summary, effective practice in working with substance misuse issues can be thought of in the words of Ashton (1999: 21):

> Be thorough; there is no substitute for quality; judge not; be welcoming and warm, but be persistent; like people and they will like you; cooperation gets the job done; help yourself by helping others; know what you should be doing, do it and do it well; explain clearly what you are up to and why; have and give confidence that together you can make things better; assume nothing. Perhaps above all – timing: catch people at the cusp of change, or somehow get them there, and the rest of the journey may be bumpy and long, but it will be down hill.

This clearly sounds more like art than science, and of course it is, but it also fits with our increased understanding of the world in which we live, and the peculiar role of human consciousness within an evolutionary environment. This then becomes the aim of our next chapter, to pull the themes together, to give us a better understanding of addictive behaviour, and to demonstrate how and why we should build upon these principles to develop our systems of interventions.

Useful resources

Egan, G. (2007) *The Skilled Helper: A Problem-management and Opportunity-Development Approach to Helping* (8th edition). Belmont, CA: Thomson Brooks/Cole.

Miller, W. and Rollnick, S. (2002) *Motivational Interviewing: Preparing People for Change* (2nd edition). New York: Guilford Press.

8

Complex Adaptive Systems: A New Paradigm for Working with Addiction?

The aims of this chapter are to:

- argue that addiction is best seen as an example of a complex self-organising system
- challenge linear and reductionist approaches to understanding and working with addiction
- discuss the application of this approach to the search for effective interventions with particular reference to motivational working.

The theme of this book is the inherently complex nature of substance use and misuse and with particular reference to the biopsychosocial paradigm. In exploring that paradigm we have taken a chronological perspective in human thinking; from the classical disease perspective, through to dependence syndromes, to psychological approaches, and then on to more recent developments in neurobiology, genomics, and evolutionary theory. It is clear that none of these disciplines is sufficient to explain drug use and addiction in isolation and all give great impetus to the important of utilising biopsychosociality for analysing, understanding, and responding to drug use and its associated problems.

It follows from this complex picture that the key challenges within the field are to build the theoretical base for understanding addictive behaviour within an interdisciplinary framework and to translate this into practical helping skills for service users and practitioners. Despite the controversies within the field (for example, about what constitutes a good outcome from interventions, the role and extent of harm reduction approaches, and the meaning of 'disease' and the extent to which individuals can regain control over their behaviour) there is some consensus that views relapse as a key feature of addiction and that addiction is 'a behaviour over which an individual has impaired control with harmful consequences' (West, 2001: 3).

It is one thing to accept that the research evidence, our experience, and 'practitioner wisdom' indicate the need for such a model of addiction, but it is quite another to deal with the implications of this at a theoretical, clinical, practical, and policy level. For example, in training professionals how much biology do social workers need to understand or how much social policy do nurses need, what should a medic's grasp of psychology be, and how does this then relate to occupational and organisational standards within services?

> Within your current course or your professional training how much emphasis has there been on issues related to substance misuse and how interdisciplinary was that approach?

Developing such a model recognises the importance of a reciprocal relationship between the individual's biological and psychological makeup, the substance, and the environment and the context in which a drug is used. Although appealing to common sense this is in itself an inherently complex proposition, given that the biology, psychology, and social context of the individual are theoretically and practically huge systems of complexity in themselves and that is before we even start to consider the interrelationships between them. The logic of the biopsychosocial paradigm is that it is about more than the sum of its individual parts (Lende and Smith, 2002) and we have seen in the previous chapters how various processes arising from genetics, neurobiology, psychology, and the social context lead to addiction. In addition, we can see that some of the negative consequences of drug use from health issues, through to psychological and social problems, may actually reinforce that problematic behaviour. It is also clear that addressing substance misuse is a major issue for society and that, despite the rhetoric of the need for more treatments, the equivalence paradox needs to be addressed. Biopsychosociality cannot simply be reduced to its component parts – the discussion on gene expression demonstrates that these are not simple and deterministic relationships, but ones in which risk factors can be increased as well as decreased through a range of other factors. Many of the insights in neurobiology have emanated from animal studies which, whilst important, with this approach may not give sufficient weight to the uniqueness of being a human animal. A part of this uniqueness takes the guise of 'culture' and for Dawkins (2006) culture is similar to genetics in that they are both transmitted and replicate themselves albeit via differing routes. From gene expression to addressing broad behavioural problems such as crime and drug use, cultural norms and mores become important because of the evidence that demonstrates issues such as stable relationships, community cohesion and employment are fundamental in overcoming these problems (see Hesselbrock and Hesselbrock, 2006; Maruna, 2001; Maruna and Immarigeon, 2004).

Our traditional approach to solving health and social problems is based upon the scientific approaches that emerged from the seventeenth century onwards and the work of Newton and Descartes. These scientific approaches very much see the world as running according to set laws which are mechanical in nature and based upon the principles of predictability, causality, reductionism, and determinism, (Cooper et al., 2008). This approach has seen an expansion of the natural, medical, and social sciences over the course of the last two centuries which has been exponential, with our crowning achievement, thus far, being the unravelling of the human genome. This knowledge, coupled with a good understanding of evolutionary theory, would it seems allow us (in the best traditions of the scientific basis of medicine) to identify a problem, make a clear diagnosis of what the problem is, and establish a method to cure the problem.

The scientific basis of treating health and health related problems has been to look for the most effective single cure. The 'Scientific Method' is the basis of modern medicine and also has a strong tradition in the social sciences. This approach is also increasingly taken by governments in seeking evidence based policies and interventions to tackle a whole range of social problems (see Pawson and Tilley, 1997; and Pawson, 2006) from clinical through to organisational practice. Particularly in the development of evidence based medicine, the randomised controlled trial (RCT) has been the gold standard of research, which seeks to demonstrate causality. The way that the RCT operates is explained by Pawson and Tilley (1997): 'identical' subjects are randomly allocated to either an experimental group or a control group, and the experimental group only are exposed to the experimental treatment. The same pre- and post-treatment measures are applied to both groups, to compare the changes in both groups. The logic of this approach is that any changes in behavioural outcome are explained by the action of the treatment and thus it is possible to infer that cause and effect are linked in a linear fashion.

One of the principles of model building in the natural and social sciences is that no model should be more complicated than it needs to be, which leads to a search for parsimonious solutions. However, as DiClemente and Prochaska (1998) point out, there are no simple solutions to complex problems and at its simplest addiction may be very complex. However, the work of Prochaska and DiClemente, and the principle of the TTM, show that there may be core processes of change which can be identified and worked with. In the preceding chapter the importance of a motivational approach was highlighted in effective working with substance misuse and in this chapter and the next we are going to look at that in more detail and suggest some implications for service provision.

As we have already seen from previous chapters, life is rarely simple and linear because of the biological, psychological, and social context in which problems arise. Within this complex framework it can be said that most issues neither have a single cause nor cure (Wilson et al., 2001). It is argued by Plsek and Greenhalgh (2001: 625) that 'across all disciplines, at all levels and throughout the world, healthcare is becoming more complex', not just in terms of the problems that people are presenting with, but also in clinical and organisational practice. This is also reflected in dealing with substance misuse problems, with the recognition of multiple needs as the norm within the 'clinical' population (see McKay and McLellan, 1998) and the need for multi-agency responses to address these issues. In 1990 the Institute of Medicine in the USA called into question whether RCTs were really the way forward in helping to address substance misuse problems and also called for a different approach to the methodology used to determine outcomes from treatment.

The need for a radical shift in the nature of the research paradigm is argued for by Orford (2008) and based upon a number of observations. In relation to equivocal outcomes from treatment he suggests that the research currently fails to address the possibility that well delivered psychological treatments (such as cognitive-behavioural therapy, motivational enhancement therapy, or Twelve Step Facilitation Therapy) are all essentially doing the same thing. In addition, given the overwhelming evidence from many service users and practitioners arguing that the therapeutic relationship is central to effective treatment, this has been an area neglected in recent research; treatment research has also failed to address the issue of unaided change, that is, change without recourse to formal treatment. This was identified by Prochaska and DiClemente in the TTM (1998) as important in building comprehensive theories of behavioural change. Orford argues that research designs to demonstrate effective outcomes have been based upon an inappropriate timescale for a chronic relapsing condition, that is, that they are too short. Measurements are usually taken at 12 months following treatments, but there are important discussions about the extensity of treatment as opposed to just the intensity of it. In addition he argues that the research agenda has been too focused upon treatment technique and has failed to take account of the broader social, familial, and circumstantial networks in which treatment is contextualised; research has privileged expert theories of treatment and very often ignored practitioners' own theories about what they are doing; and in the same vein the role of service users in treatment research has been a passive one of providing data rather than actively contributing to an understanding of the change process. Finally, Orford would say that whilst in social science generally there has been an increasing amount of critique of scientific method, particularly in relation to notions of causality and linear relationships, this has not been the case in the field of addictions, where the randomised controlled trial is still seen as the gold standard of research.

Complexity Theory

Complexity Theory is a discipline that has arisen from Chaos Theory and the study of complex dynamics in the physical sciences, economics, and the social sciences (Holder, 1999). What this approach demonstrates is that 'chaotic' and 'random' behaviour occurs naturally within deterministic systems (in this sense chaos is not the absence of rules but the outcomes from those rules) precisely because the nature of these systems is one of non-linearity. It is this non-linearity which is the key to understanding complexity and refers to the fact that input into a system is not necessarily proportionate to output. It might be argued, for example, that the more severe a substance misuse problem is in terms of dependence and the problems involved the more frequent and intensive 'treatment' is required than for someone with a less severe problem. However, on the basis of relapse rates, equivalence, and also paradoxical outcomes (see Miller, 2006) we know that this approach is not necessarily correct. Complexity demonstrates that minor changes in a system can cause massive changes to the structure and dynamics of that system, which would not be predictable simply by observing the component parts (the approach used by the RCT). Complex systems are by nature adaptive and transformational and this understanding has led to the study of Complex Adaptive Systems (CAS) of which addiction is increasingly being seen as an example (Bickel and Potenza, 2006: see below).

In addition to non-linearity the other key concept within complexity is that of self-organisation or 'order for free' (Kaufman, 1993, cited by Bickell and Potenza, 2006). This is a process which increases the organisation of a system without the help of an external designer and is ubiquitous within Darwinian biology, occuring in every system composed of inter-connected elements. The use of cellula automata below demonstrates this in action.

Complexity Theory provides us with a useful set of tools with which to understand the nature of the ways in which multi-agented systems such as the biopsychosocial system of addiction operate. This approach raises important questions about the nature of interaction effects, whether the perceived solutions are a part of the problem, the nature of emergent prop-erties, or the role of randomness. This then challenges us to develop appro-priate ethical responses to those issues based upon our understanding of them. Importantly, this approach takes into account an increased under-standing of the ways in which a system evolves and adapts. In terms of theory building and its application to practice this becomes an important step in identifying the nature of effective interventions, how we define and operate them, and what we think the outcomes from them should be. In addition, this approach allows us to develop our new insights into evolution-ary theory as well, and on this basis Bar-Yam (1997: 5) has stated that, 'The study of complex systems in a unified framework has become recognised… as … the ultimate in interdisciplinary fields'.

A busy practitioner, or a policy maker, or a commissioner of services, could well ask whether it is necessary to take thinking around drug use and addiction to such a level of abstraction. The response would be that complexity theory provides us with a whole systems approach that has the potential to offer higher order solutions to complex problems. Moreover, it is vitally important that theory informs practice and that our practice is based upon ethical considerations of what we know to be the cause of a particular problem or set of problems. In addition, by utilising a new para-digm such as that of viewing addiction as an example of a complex adaptive system this can then provide new insights and opportunities for practitioners and service users alike.

Complex Adaptive Systems (CAS)

A complex adaptive system is defined as 'a collection of individual agents with freedom to act in ways that are not always totally predictable, and whose actions are interconnected so that the action of one part changes the context for other agents' (Wilson et al., 2001: 685). Human Beings, communities, families, eco-systems and governments are all of examples of complex systems, and Bar-Yam (1997) outlines the elements that distinguish them from simple systems. These include the number of elements involved, and subsequent interactions between those elements and their strength, the formation and operation of the system and the timescales involved, the diversity and variability of the system, the environment in which it exists and the demands that it places upon the system, as well as the activities and objectives of that system.

The key properties of complex adaptive systems are outlined by Holt (2004): a CAS is a multi-agented system that is connected through local agent–agent interactions which tend to be non-linear and feedback on each other; the boundaries between the internal agents and the system and its environment are indistinct and dynamic; energy and other resources are taken from the environment and are continuously dissipated, keeping the system far from equilibrium, and although there is a turnover of components, structure and information are preserved over time; importantly the system can adapt to changes in the internal and external environment and there is an overlap between sub-categories of agent in the system so that an individual may belong to more than one sub-category; because of this connectivity, the existence of fuzzy boundaries and overlap, it is difficult to simply remove a part of the system and replace it; the system has a history which determines its current structure, internal organisation and behaviour, so that it is capable of learning; emergent properties may arise through the lower level interactions between agents and such properties cannot be understood at the level of the agents themselves (that is, the sum is more than the total of the parts).

In relation to human health and functioning the following levels of complex adaptive systems can be identified; for these reasons Wilson, Holt and Greenhalgh (2001) argue that human behaviour is unpredictable and cannot simply be modelled in a cause and effect manner.

- The human body is composed of multiple interacting and self-regulating physiological systems (such as 'homeostasis' as outlined in Chapter 6).
- Individual behaviour is determined partly by internal rules developed through past experience (see the discussion on social learning and conditioning in Chapter 5) and partly by unique and adaptive responses to new stimuli from the environment (see the discussion on evolutionary theory in Chapter 6).
- The web of relationships in which individuals exist may powerfully determine beliefs, expectations and behaviours (consider the role of social context and peer pressure in relation to substance use).
- These immediate social circumstances are further embedded in wider social, political and cultural systems which can influence outcomes in unpredictable ways (consider the way that the supply and availability of psychoactive substances are legislated for).

- Interacting systems are dynamic and fluid (it would appear that some people may move in and out of problematic substance use and addiction).
- Small changes in one part of the system can lead to much larger changes in another part of the system (one drink or use of a drug can lead to a major relapse or not).

Thus an understanding of complexity is to move away from the idea of linear relationships with singular causes, to a focus on decentralised interactions and feedback loops, which emerge from simple interactions. Importantly CAS are modular in nature and are made up of sub-systems or modules (similar to modern computers), so that there is no overall control mechanism, which means that if one part of the system fails, then another part compensates for it, meaning that there is not a wholesale incapacitation of the system. It can be seen that within an evolutionary context these systems are dynamic and adaptable in nature and demonstrate emergent properties.

Recapping Complex Adaptive Systems (Bickell and Potenza, 2006)

Within CAS 'complexity' refers to the multiple elements, levels, interactions, and sub-systems which are continually operating within the system; 'adaptation' refers to the system's ability to accommodate perturbations (threats) from within or outside the system and is a feature that is fundamental to all living organisms and social structures; 'dynamic' refers to a system's inherent drive to change (and survive) through the constant interactions of its lower order components; 'emergent properties' demonstrate that the whole is greater than the sum of its parts; and 'homeostasis' shows that the system may exist as a sub-optimal level and is 'locked in' through a variety of feeback loops.

Cellular Automata

A useful and straightforward way to model the behaviour of these interaction effects is through the use of Cellular Automata (Guastello and Liebovitch, 2009). We do not need to concern ourselves too much with the theory and maths of this, except to say that Cellular Automata (CA) are a collection of cells (normally coloured) placed on a grid, that evolve through a series of time steps. (More information about Cellular Automata can be found at http://mathworld.wolfram.com.)

In addition to having a position on a grid, the cell has a 'neighbourhood' which it affects and is itself affected by other cells depending upon some basic rules of 'engagement'. Below (Diagram 1) is a simplified use of CA that demonstrates the key qualities of a complex system emerging from simple interactions and which also show evolutionary (emergent), dynamic and adaptable behaviour. In this model the rules of interaction are as follows.

- A cell remains alive with two or three contiguous neighbours.
- A cell dies of overcrowding with more than three neighbours.
- A cell dies of exposure with less than two live neighbours.
- An empty cell becomes alive if three neighbouring cells are alive.
- All the moves are synchronous.

Diagram 1 **Cellular Automata**

	1	2	3	4	5	6	7	8
2								
3				X		X		
4				X	X			
5						X		
6								
7								
8								

Time Step One

	1	2	3	4	5	6	7	8
2								
3				X	X			
4				X	X			
5								
6								
7								
8								

Time Step Two

	1	2	3	4	5	6	7	8
1								
2								
3			X	X	X			
4			X		X			
5								
6								
7								
8								

Time Step Three

	1	2	3	4	5	6	7	8
1								
2				X				
3			X	X	X			
4			X	X	X			
5								
6								
7								
8								

Time Step Four

	1	2	3	4	5	6	7	8
1								
2			X	X	X			
3			X		X			
4			X		X			
5								
6								
7								
8								

Time Step Five

1	2	3	4	5	6	7	8
2							
3							
4		X	X	X			
5		X		X			
6							
7							
8							

Time Step Six

1	2	3	4	5	6	7	8
2							
3			X				
4		X	X	X			
5		X	X	X			
6							
7							
8							

In this example the number of elements and the original position on the graph were completely chosen at random and have produced a system that has become 'locked in' from Time Step Three; it will simply continue as it is infinitely.

> Practise creating your own systems of CA and see how they grow and develop. Recognise which ones last and which ones become extinct.

Intervention effects

Using this approach it is interesting to see what happens when variables are introduced that are intended to disrupt the system (see Diagram 2), in the same way that an intervention is used to tackle substance misuse problems (the white Xs are the interventions). What are important are the interaction effects between all of the variables including the intervention, so that the intervention has to be seen as a part of the problem as well as the potential solution. Another random system has been plotted on the grid, but this time the rules of engagement are:

- A cell remains alive with two or three contiguous neighbours and no contiguous intervention.
- A cell dies of overcrowding with more than two neighbours and an intervention.
- A cell dies from exposure if there are less than two live neighbours.
- An empty cell becomes alive if there are three neighbouring cells and no contiguous intervention.
- As before all of the moves are synchronous.
- For the purposes of this exercise the 'interventions' are not dependent upon the system that it is addressing to 'stay alive', it has a life independent of the system.

Diagram 2   **Cellular Automata with Intervention**

1	2	3	4	5	6	7	8
2							
3							
4							
5						X	X
6					X	X	
7				X		X	
8					X		

Time Step One

1	2	3	4	5	6	7	8
2							
3							
4							
5							
6							X
7				X	X		
8					X		

Time Step Two

1	2	3	4	5	6	7	8
2							
3							
4							
5							
6							
7				X	X		
8				X	X		

From this example it can be seen that the 'interventions' do in fact disrupt the system, but importantly that the system adapts, responds to the threat, and moves away from the intervention. It is clear that the more robust the system is in having more variables interacting with each other then potentially, as you try to address the problem, the more opportunity there is for emergent issues to occur.

All we are trying to do here is to model interaction effects and some of the behaviours of complex adaptive systems and particularly to highlight the importance of the system being dynamic, adaptive, and evolutionary in nature. We can use this as a kind of metaphor to help in conceptualising the nature of the problem. Although this abstract model tells us nothing about temporal relations in the real world, it does summarise systems effects and also highlights the importance of where and how interventions are positioned, their extensiveness, and whether there is a need for a multimodal approach (McGuire, 1995). If you use this approach with more intervention variables and position them in and around the system, it is interesting to see the extent to which the system can adapt and survive.

> Experiment with 'intervention' variables to see what impact their positioning has on the system.

Motivational working restated

William Miller (2006: 149) states that 'once substance abuse/dependence has been established, education, persuasion, confrontation, punishment and attention typically yield little or no beneficial effect and sometimes exert a paradoxical effect'. He also makes the point that if punishment is the imposition of a negative consequence to a particular behaviour (i.e. drug taking) then because of the negative consequences associated with drug taking that occurs anyway we would expect this kind of behaviour to be very uncommon. This is an important issue in relation to contemporary treatment practice in the UK, where coerced interventions via the criminal justice system have grown exponentially but without visible benefit (see below). However, the issue here is the way in which organisms and systems respond to threats through the flight or fight mechanism (Gardner, 2009) to ensure their survival. Any system that is intended to help individuals, including psychotherapeutic talking therapies, has to ensure that it is not perceived as a threat; hence the importance of the worker–service user relationship based upon empathic principles.

The challenges to this empathic approach arise within the context of workers providing a range of functions at the same time as including that of making a diagnosis, providing emotional and practical support, keeping notes, and meeting occupational and organisational standards, to name just a few (see Pincus, 2009). Pincus (2009: 336) argues that 'Therapists are pulled by competing biopsychosocial forces … as they attempt to stay present and aware of these processes, within the client, within themselves, and among the two'. This also highlights the importance of good professional supervision for people working with these kinds of issues. But one of the main challenges to an effective approach for addressing substance misuse problems stems from the use of coerced interventions.

The role of coercion

Seddon (2007) outlines the rationale for coerced treatment within the criminal justice system, particularly the view that there is a strong causal relationship between addiction and acquisitive crime, that treatment is effective in reducing 'drug-related' crime. He looks at the idea of 'coercion' as trying to persuade someone to do something they are unwilling to do through the use of force or threats and which is contrasted with voluntary treatment. The policy issues related to this increased use of coerced treatments are summarised by Reuter and Stevens (2008) who demonstrate that the number of people entering treatment via a court order has risen from 1,886 in 1995 to 11,286 in 2006, and that these figures do not include entry to treatment via the criminal justice system but without a court order. Likewise within the Probation Service, the Offender Management Caseload Statistics (Home Office, 2007) show that the number of probation commencements including an order for drug treatment more than doubled from 5,855 in 2005 to 12,145 in 2007; for alcohol this nearly tripled from 1,356 in 2005 to 3,267 in 2007. This was prior to the national roll out of the Alcohol Treatment Requirement and so the number of orders for alcohol treatment will increase still further. However, according to Reuter and Stevens (2008), despite the huge investment in drug services in the criminal justice system, this has had very little impact upon overall crime rates. This approach to treatment is a classic example of linear thinking – more treatment equals better outcomes – but it is quite clear that the nature of that treatment is fundamental to the kinds of outcomes that can be expected.

With an increased emphasis by New Labour on law and order issues, and the development of a whole range of interventions which can be accessed via the criminal justice system, then more and more agencies and professionals have to work with and alongside the criminal justice system. The difficulty here is that the approach the criminal justice system takes would appear to be completely at odds with what we know the nature of addiction to be.

Rational actors?

The approach of the criminal justice system is to treat people as rational actors who choose to commit crimes and are therefore morally responsible for their actions. As a consequence of ignoring alternative possibilities of action (see Widerker and McKenna, 2006), offenders are deemed deserving of punishment in the form of society taking retribution and also in the hope of deterring others from doing the same thing. The difficulty here is that although drug use may initially involve choice, when that use becomes 'addictive behaviour' we are faced with a system of impaired control and relapse as a centrally defining feature. Within this complex biopsychosocial paradigm responsibility becomes an aspiration and not a given; it is something that we all work towards and at times struggle with. If a person has a problems such as addiction and is seeking to overcome it, then like any major change in life it is something that may take time and require encouragement rather than condemnation. This is the basis of Motivational Interviewing. The key features of coerced interventions tend to involve being tested on a regular basis and if the test is positive for drug use then the person is sent back to court with the risk of a custodial sentence being imposed. Given that relapse is a defining feature of addiction the fundamental question becomes this: are we simply setting people up to fail?

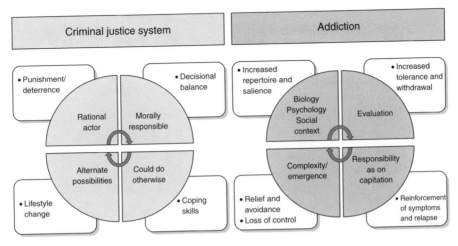

FIGURE 8.1 *Criminal justice and addiction as systems of coercion*

It is interesting when considering the nature of addiction and the growth of criminal justice responses to it to compare and contrast the nature of the two systems and see them both as systems of coercion albeit with differing 'intentions'.

In Figure 8.1 I have overlaid the criminal justice–rational actor model with a standard CBT approach concerned with decision making and coping skills. This stands in contrast to the key features of dependence syndromes but is underpinned by our understanding of the evolutionary and complex nature of addiction. This stands in contrast with what we know about the nature of addiction, the realities of relapse, and its emergent properties.

Through complexity, compulsion, and impaired control the system of addiction in reality reduces the number of alternate possibilities that an individual feels they have. A great deal of focus and energy is on dealing with the system's drive to survive. In contrast the criminal justice system through promoting the value of retributive deterrence seeks to coerce drug users into treatment and to provide opportunities for treatment (see Figure 8.2). Again it promises alternate possibilities without taking into account the true nature of the problem.

A new paradigm

Within the framework of complexity theory drug problems are the natural outputs of dynamic, complex, and adaptive systems that we call

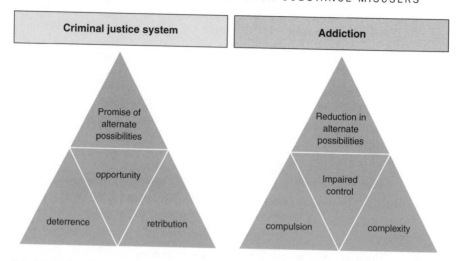

FIGURE 8.2   *Methods of coercion by systems of criminal justice and addiction*

'communities' and Holder (1999) argues that if we only work with the high risk individuals to gain short term reductions in problems then the system will simply adapt to accommodate those changes. This approach shows that interventions do not always yield the desired effects and that prevention strategies to be successful have to try and alter the system that produces the problems. Within prevention approaches, strategies have tended to focus on single solutions rather than concurrent reinforcing approaches (Holder, 1999).

Within this framework prevention strategies are important and in rela-tion to psychoactive substances none more so than the control of their supply and availability. As we have seen in previous chapters the most com-pelling information is in relation to alcohol, with comparative data show-ing the correlation between consumption and problems. A similar argument can be made for illicit drugs: that a huge investment in the dis-ruption of drug markets has meant that the number of Class A drug users in the UK is only at about 300,000. In debates about the legalisation and decriminalisation of certain drugs, one feature is that the numbers of users would increase.

Prevention strategies can never be perfect, not least because the 'Pursuit of Oblivion' (Davenport-Hines, 2001; 2004) has been a long term human endeavour and as a consequence of occurring within an evolutionary environment has affected our genetic make up. The important questions then revolve around what to do with someone once they have developed an addiction to a substance. Everything that we have looked at within the nature of the problem tells us that we need to view this from a chronic disease perspective, one that views the problem over a time course and works with the motivation of the individual concerned. This time course will involve a relapse and often multiple relapses, in which problems will be resolved and new problems will emerge. Within this process medication can play an important role, either as a substitute for a drug or as an adjunct to talking therapies. The choice of therapy should come down to the service user themselves, with the importance being on the way that the therapy is delivered and by whom. Are the organisation and its representatives acting as agents of hope, working with motivational approaches? Are any interacting needs of relationships, employment, housing, and education being addressed to ensure that the system that has contributed to the maintenance of the substance misuse problem is being taken into account?

Theory of Mind

Finally the emphasis has been on empathic non-threatening relationships as an effective way of working with complex interacting problems such as addiction. The nature of this relationship which has been developed by Carl Rogers is cited by Miller and Rollnick (2002) as accurate empathy, non-possessive warmth, and being genuine. In describing accurate empathy they warn that this should not be confused with identifying with a person or as having similar experiences, as this can in fact compromise the relationship through an over-identification with the problems involved. This is an interesting point because many rehabilitation organisations in the substance misuse field deliberately employ graduates of their programmes as counsellors and workers because of their understanding of the issues. For Miller and Rollnick (2002: 7) (and building on the work of Carl Rogers) 'accurate empathy involves skilful reflective listening that clarifies and amplifies the person's own experiencing and meaning, without imposing the counsellor's own material'.

This approach is in keeping with our understanding of the development of the brain and social communication within an evolutionary context. One of the arguments from evolutionary psychology is that the brain should not be considered as a general purpose computer designed to solve any problem, but rather as having developed in a modular way to address specific adaptive problems (Bickell and Potenza, 2006). Within a Darwinian context the brain needs to address the environmental uncertainty and threat to the individual to ensure survival, to be able to weigh up, compete with, and triumph over others (Braithwaite et al., 2007). In recent years this has led to the study of a concept know as 'Theory of Mind' and refers to the ability of people to understand and predict the behaviour of others as well as their knowledge, intentions, emotions, and beliefs (Tirapu-Ustarroz et al., 2007).

Theory of mind originated in the study of autism, but has recently developed within the areas of schizophrenia and psychoses. Having a theory of mind means that we believe other people have minds like our own and so we can understand their behaviour in terms of the contents of their minds (Frith, 2004). Frith goes onto argue that someone who does not have a theory of mind takes no account of other people's beliefs and desires when trying to understand their behaviour. In respect of working with others through the use of interpersonal skills, Ratcliffe and Hutto (2007: 1) suggest that 'the concepts that we employ to interpret and interact with people will be closely related to, if not the same as, the concepts that constitute our sense of what people are'. In professional helping settings it is important that this moves beyond common sense to intuitive responses to people's problems, with applications that have coherence, validity, and accountability as well.

There is a growing literature on theory of mind which may offer us important insights into our understanding of human relationships and the specific relationships that are required to meet helping and counselling functions. What theory of mind demonstrates is the importance of mental states, non-verbal behaviour, and the role of language. Within this context the importance of empathy is stressed (see Saxe and Baron-Cohen, 2006) and it may be that when faced with a problem as dynamic, adaptable, and as complex as addiction that only the human brain and personality is able to keep pace with that system to effect change.

Useful resources

Guastello, S.J., Koopmans, M. and Pincus, D. (eds) (2009) *Chaos and Complexity in Psychology*. Cambridge: Cambridge University Press.

Holder, H. (1999) *Alcohol and the Community: A Systems Approach to Prevention*. Cambridge: Cambridge University Press.

Holt, T. (ed.) (2004) *Complexity for Clinicians*. Oxford: Radcliffe.

9

Pulling it all Together: An Extended Case Study

The aims of this chapter are, through the use of an extended case study, to:

- highlight the key themes raised in the book with respect to the biopsychosocial paradigm
- highlight particularly issues concerning evolution, emergence, and adaptation
- encourage reflection upon those key themes.

The following interview was carried out specifically as a case study for this book, and at her request, apart from her first name, Fiona remains entirely anonymous. My meeting with Fiona was entirely serendipitous; the peer review for this book had requested a case study and a real life example emerged after a meeting at an academic conference. Apart from polishing some of the dialogue in terms of removing 'ers' and 'ums' the account is verbatim (it was digitally recorded and professionally transcribed). It is worth reading the account a couple of times to become familiar with the themes and also I would make the point that we covered a great deal of ground in one hour. I present the interview in a way that allows Fiona to speak for herself in responding to my questions and although she is willing to be very open about her experiences it is important to remember that it is also an account of a very traumatic life; as such there is a great deal of information but this should not be seen as a complete biography. In giving the account there will obviously be gaps to be filled and other questions to be answered.

On reading the case study and engaging with the interview the reader is encouraged to look for evidence for some of the themes covered in this book and to reflect upon them in the following way:

What is the evidence in this case study for the following in leading to, and maintaining, addictive behaviour:

Biology (see Chapters 3, 5 and 6)

- Evolutionary processes including genetics and the dis-regulation of the CMDA in impairing motivation and creating multiple problem areas including poly drug use?
- What is the evidence for physical and mental health problems associated with drug use?

Psychology (see Chapters 5, 7, and 8)

- The role of motivation, self-efficacy, and self-esteem?
- Modelling other people's behaviours?
- The importance of decision making and behavioural outcomes?
- Concurrent mental health problems?

Social context (see Chapters 1, 2, 5, 6, 7, 8)

- The importance of family background?
- The role of other personal relationships?
- The supply and availability of drugs?
- The impact of trauma?
- Access to material resources?
- The role of coercion?

Emergent properties (see Chapters 7 and 8)

- Addiction as a dynamic system made up of interacting parts, which survives through adaptation and responding to threats (perturbations)?

What is the evidence for the following in overcoming addictive behaviour:
Interventions (see Chapters 3, 4, 5, 7 and 8)

- The role of motivation?
- The role of coercion?
- Decision making leading to actions and changes in behaviours?
- The maintenance of those changes?
- The role of relapse?
- Resources available from statutory and non-statutory agencies?
- The role of self-help?
- Key features of the support available and the people involved?
- A Recovery Meme?

THE CASE STUDY

Aaron: I suppose what would be useful for a start would be to know a little bit about you, and your context in terms of your experience of having an alcohol problem.

Fiona: And drugs that's the bit that not many people are aware of but that does feature somewhat largely at points.

Aaron: OK so it would be useful to try and put some kind of framework around your experience in terms of complexity. So in that respect my key words are, complexity, adaptation, dynamic, emergent properties, and homeostasis and so on ...

Fiona: I first tried to get sober when I was 17 because I'd – I started drinking very early so probably round about by 12, 13, drinking was a problem. It was definitely a problem by the time I was 17, so, at that point I then didn't drink for two years.

Aaron: From 17?

Fiona: To 19. But with no awareness of what the problem was, no help, no nothing, obviously that two years was a bit miserable really. So I went off to University in Leeds and started drinking again. So that was, um, right up until 1998 when I was 40 when I got into recovery.

Aaron: So you were drinking heavily through university?

Fiona: Yes.

Aaron: All the way up until you were 40 or ...?

Fiona: Yeah.

Aaron: Did you try and get sober at any points during that time?

Fiona: The only time I did was ... well, there's a lot of stuff that goes before this and around it.

Aaron: Okay.

Fiona: As you're probably aware because you don't just say, right do you know today I'm going to start drinking, it didn't happen like that. What do I think causes alcoholism is part of the question really I think that you were asking ... so I was adopted, when I was about three and a half months old, into a family where my mother – or – adoptive mother had – Munchausen's by proxy and my father was – or adoptive father was – sexually abusive. My adoptive elder brother, was also adopted in the family, so none of us were related, if you see what I mean, I think he didn't have a good time because he was very violent as well. So there was a lot of stuff went on in the family, perhaps that's the reason I picked up and started drinking so early, I don't know.

Aaron: You don't know?

Fiona: However, in 2001 I met my real family; mother, father, two brothers, two sisters, all practising alcoholics.

(Continued)

(Continued)

Aaron: Okay so, there's a strong genetic link?

Fiona: There is. There is obviously, but I'm out of the debating society because I don't care what caused it. But certainly it was no surprise to me when I met my family – and I don't see them any more because it's pointless. I'm sober, they're not. They don't like my sobriety, I can't take their drinking, it's just not going to happen, do you know what I mean, so ...

Aaron: So what you paint straightaway is, is a very complex picture, and I think what you're saying is it's very difficult to say, right, this is what causes ... me to kind of drink heavily. But if you were to start to identify what you think the key influences were on your drinking what would you identify? I mean was there for example other drinking going on in your adoptive family?

Fiona: No.

Aaron: Or in your peer group?

Fiona: No. So that was interesting, my drinking was always abnormal.

Aaron: Right, within your context it was abnormal?

Fiona: Yeah. So by the age of 17 my drinking had caused me so many problems that I knew drinking was causing a problem, so I stopped drinking for that two years, I was almost 20 and I tried to commit suicide, at the end of the two years of not drinking. So obviously the drinking helped with what had been going on in the family, but that two years was just hellish and I didn't want to drink and I didn't really want to live with the family, so it seemed the ideal solution ... and so I was on life support for six days, it was, it was, um, a very serious attempt, and I can remember coming round and thinking, God I didn't want to be there. But I started drinking immediately I came of the hospital, so that, the upshot of that was really that the drinking just carried on from there, so no attempt to get sober at all. But I didn't know I had a problem.

Aaron: That's interesting I'll come back to that, but I mean in terms of your drinking behaviour, did you also have other mental health issues as well?

Fiona: Looking back I would say very definitely, very definitely, but it's hard to say where those ... what were actually mental health issues and what were survival techniques ... Because obviously with my mother's problem, constantly ill, always in the hospital with broken bones, all that sort of thing, having to lie about all of those things that happened ... So I think, yeah, mental health issues definitely by the time I'd finished drinking, in my early days it's really difficult looking back because it was so confused. Because what then happened was I went off and I did my university then joined the air force as a commissioned officer. And I had a car accident in 1981 and I broke my neck but I'd completely lost the use of my left arm, and for years that was, that was sort of seen as nerve damage ... I had another accident in the States, and I went to see a neurologist, and they thought to do a brain scan and it was actually brain damage. Well, they think that the brain damage was caused from what had been going on in the home, and the car accident was the, the final straw that caused it. I don't know if you've heard of it but its caused Dystonia? So I was paralysed down my left-hand side for 19 years.

Aaron: So when you started drinking at 12 or 13 ... was it, a conscious choice to start drinking?

Fiona: Do you know there were stories that were really quite famous within the family that when I was two I managed to pick up a glass of sherry and I downed it in one, giggled a lot, and then they had to hide any drink from me after that, if ever I got hold of drink I'd just down it, which I always did, I mean it never made sense to me until I got sober and I thought, oh, perhaps those were some early indications. Do you know, I can't remember.

Aaron: So violence within the adoptive home and sexual abuse? Was that something that the, the whole family was aware of, or was it just, your adoptive father?

Fiona: I have no idea looking back, they were completely odd, the whole family was odd, how much of it got outside the home I don't know. Certainly my brothers never talked about it, erm, my adoptive brother, but we've never been close, but ... when my adoptive mother died in 1999, because they lived in Yorkshire – I went up there, and he looked at me and he said, I'll go to the funeral and if anybody ever mentions that name to me again they're out of the house and I'll never speak to them again. So I'm ... I can only assume that he was subject to, to the same things, but obviously he wasn't going to talk about it.

Fiona: His behaviour was very violent not just to me ...

Aaron: Okay. So, I suppose what I'm interested in from the age of 12, 13 onwards – was whether there were variations in your drinking or, or if there was a drinking pattern whether it developed over the course of that time.

Fiona: Up until 17?

Aaron: Yes.

Fiona: Do you know, I've never really thought about it. I suppose it was all really at the weekends.

Aaron: Like binge drinking?

Fiona: Yeah. Yeah. Very much like, like the binge drinkers are now, that, you know, I'd look forward to a weekend and look forward to drinking. Obviously I was so young that even my friends were not interested in what I was doing, they didn't want to be involved, and so a lot of it was very secretive.

Aaron: So presumably by the time you were 17 you were drinking to an extent that you were concerned?

(Continued)

(Continued)

Fiona: That I was in trouble, yes.

Aaron: Okay. And how would you know that? What were the signs ... ?

Fiona :   I was working as a waitress, I got sacked from that job, my parents
          weren't really, speaking to me, there was just silence in the house all
          the time, um, sexually promiscuous – which I didn't want to be but
          didn't seem to be able to, to stop – every time I had a drink, um, and
          that's why the ... I stopped drinking, really.

Aaron: So it sounds like, you were in quite a lot of conflict and ambivalence
          around what you're doing knowing actually you needed to do
          something ... but not knowing what to do ... or how to go about it? So
          going to what you said earlier, did your, adoptive parents try to help
          you to get help?

Fiona: No not at all. I think they were concerned that if anything ever went
          outside the family that all the rest ... you know, this is only in hindsight
          but at the time it was always said that if we ever spoke about my
          mother's problem we would die, you know, and I spent a lot of my
          childhood and early years in fear of being killed ... from saying anything.
          But the sexual abuse actually stopped round about when I was 11,
          because I got myself – looking back how sad is this – a 40-year-old
          boyfriend and told my father that he was now my boyfriend and if my
          father did anything ever again he'd kill him.

Fiona: Sad, isn't it?

Aaron: Sad, or ... sounds quite brave as well ... a statement of strength.

Aaron: So when you first tried to get sober what ... who did you go to for help?

Fiona: I just did everything on my own. I became very much an own person,
          you know, everything I did I had to do on my own. When I went to
          university my parents wouldn't give me any money to go so I worked
          my way through, I became very self-sufficient very early. So I just
          stopped drinking, made a decision but I didn't change any other
          behaviour. I wasn't sexually promiscuous any more but I still went to
          the pub with everybody, and felt even more out of things than I had
          when I was drinking.

Aaron: Was it just drinking at that stage or was it drugs?

Fiona: No, just drinking. I was incredibly anti-drugs at that stage.

Aaron: Do you think there are kind of similarities between your sexual behaviour
          and your drinking as well?

Fiona: Yes, absolutely.

Aaron: So, I mean, is it too strong to suggest that they were both an addiction?

Fiona: Yes, I would say so. And what happened from the age of 17, my new
          addiction was sport, keep fit, aerobics.

Aaron: Okay but still drinking?

Fiona: No, at 17 to 19 I didn't drink. So at that stage I was incredibly fit,
          every spare minute was spent doing some form of exercise, going to
          an exercise class.

Aaron: And then you went to university? And started drinking again?

Fiona: Yeah.

Aaron: And why was that, do you think ... ?

Fiona: Because I didn't want to feel left out. All the social life was down the pub. So I wanted to be part of that.

Aaron: At what point did drugs come into it? Was that at university or was that after? And when we're talking about drugs are we talking about illegal drugs or prescribed drugs?

Fiona: Well, it started off with prescribed drugs, it started off, when I had, my car accident, I did actually break my neck and so I was given really heavy painkillers and I was on traction for months, and loads of operations, all that sort of thing, so it was blagging as many prescription drugs as I could get, along with alcohol. I was in the air force at that time and the station commander used to come and see me with a few of his buddies, they were searched on the way in to make sure that they hadn't brought me any alcohol. And that never struck me as significant obviously, but I would, I'd get people to try and bring in alcohol any way that I could.

Aaron: It was a recognised problem?

Fiona: By everybody else.

Aaron: By everybody else ... except you?

Fiona: Yeah.

Aaron: So you started drinking again at 19 ...

Fiona: Yes.

Aaron: So did you start drinking where you'd left off or was it getting kind of progressively worse?

Fiona: It got worse very, very quickly. Because it was drinking during the week then, but that was okay because I was a student. So whereas other people would go to one event during the week I'd have all sorts of events during the week and do it, do it that way so that I could drink every day.

Aaron: Okay so looking back was your drinking a problem at that stage?

Fiona: It was always a problem, whenever I drank it was a problem.

Aaron: So was it impacting on your studies?

Fiona: I'd always been a high achiever, this, this was part of my problem, I didn't really have to work ... to get an average score. So, no, it didn't. So I could behave the way I wanted, go to the odd lecture, read the notes and, and pass the exams.

Aaron: So there were no real indications at the time that you needed to change behaviour?

Fiona: No. Apart from the fact everybody thought I was just wild. I was just, you know, the one, it used to be if Fiona's there you've got a party, and I suppose I quite liked that as a reputation.

Aaron: It sounds as of you were then drinking constantly for a number of years?

(Continued)

(Continued)

Fiona: Yes.

Aaron: Constantly and consistently? Were there points – I suppose it's an obvious question really, but, you know, what other kind of issues or problems emerged during the course of that time? Because I mean you talked about having the car accidents and, other things, would you put all those, put those down to the drinking?

Fiona: If I'm honest, yes. The first one I was the driver, we were at home, it was about 11 o'clock Sunday morning and I'd had a large sherry before we went out so, yes, I'd say that was possibly the case. The, the other thing I should say is that I was also anorexic. So when I came into recovery I was two and a half stone lighter than I am now, so it didn't take a lot with me really to get drunk.

Aaron: And did your drinking pattern stay the same ... were you an everyday drinker, did you keep yourself topped up?

Fiona: Yeah. I was an everyday drinker. That ... at the height of my drinking, apart from the last year, at the height of my drinking the maximum amount I ever drank was a bottle a day, of wine. That doesn't sound a lot, but for somebody who's five and a half stone it was ... and it, it wasn't really the amount I drank it was what happened when I drank.

Aaron: Were there other problems that emerged when you drank?

Fiona: Yeah, I think so, I left home to join the air force and that was an escape. Well, I was offered a place at Cambridge but, my father was desperate for me to go there, so I thought, well, I won't do that. So I joined the air force instead. So this is just, patterns of stuff, and I thought the air force would be a brilliant escape, but it wasn't because he quite liked the idea of that once I was commissioned and I was an officer. So then I got married to somebody he didn't like but I'd basically married my father ... so that was a very violent marriage ... the reason I'm talking about that in context with the drink is because it was easier to stay than to go.

Fiona: And what I used to do with my life was to say to people, oh, here you are, here's my life, you take responsibility for it and I'll just go off and do what I want. So despite the fact I was being beaten up all the time here was somebody who paid the bills, and all that sort of thing. So what I then did was I took jobs that took me around the world where I didn't have to be at home, because my drinking was now being remarked upon ... in the marital home. So rather than stop drinking what I did was move myself out of the marital home Monday to Friday.

Aaron: So that's a nice example of a kind of adaptation to the ... perceived threat to your drinking?

Fiona: Yes.

Aaron: So you changed what you were doing?

Fiona: Yeah. Yeah.

Fiona: What's really interesting is that man was eventually arrested and taken away for trying to kill me, so I knew there was always a threat

	on my life, that didn't matter, I'd stay with the marriage, but you threaten my drinking and I did something about it.
Aaron:	I mean you have already used the term, but do you describe yourself as an alcoholic?
Fiona:	Mm-hm.
Aaron:	Would you say that you've always been an alcoholic?
Fiona:	Yes.
Aaron:	So right back, you know, so the stories of you being two or three and drinking sherry … ?
Fiona:	Yeah. I met about, ten years ago, somebody I'd been at school with, and I hadn't seen her since, oh, God, I was about 20, and she said, do you know, she said, there was always something about you and drinking, even when we were really, really young, and it was, it was obsessive, it was pick up a drink and get drunk, every time, there was nothing … I would rather not have a drink than have one drink.
Aaron:	You just wanted to drink to get drunk?
Fiona:	Yes.
Aaron:	Okay. So what was your experience of trying to get sober?
Fiona:	That was really interesting, I'll just go through the bit of the story because it's all interleaved, talking about complexity. So I was in this violent marriage, doing these jobs that went, all over the place, and in the end I knew that in order to save my own life I had to leave and so I went out and I got a job in America but I didn't tell him until I'd got there. Rang him up and said, look, I'm working in America now, I'm not coming home, which seeing as he'd seen me leave for work that morning it was a bit of a shock, so I lived in America for a year and a half, and it was in America that I really got involved in street drugs. So leading up to that I'd been … I'd had all these painkillers, got lots of painkillers, then I went to the States and got involved with a group, during the week that, took cocaine every day. Fine. Didn't drink during the week. At the weekends I had a group of friends who drank, didn't take drugs. So in my head I wasn't a drug addict because I didn't take drugs at the weekend, and not an alchie because I didn't drink during the week. So this was a cycle that grew, and I came home from the States, got divorced, and bought a house. Now this was all doing stuff to change, so the geographical to America, coming home, another geographical, hoping that it would mend things, bought the house, that worked for a while. I think I got a dog somewhere in there as well. Then I decided that I needed to get pregnant because that would, that would be the thing that would mend my life completely. But I was taking a drug that was a wonderful mixture of morphine, valium and something else. But they said to me, whilst I was taking this drug not to get pregnant. So I completely ignored all of that. Didn't have a boyfriend and I knew I needed one if I was going to achieve this ambition. So got one boyfriend, thought that might not

(Continued)

(Continued)

be enough so I got two and ended up getting pregnant. But at 20 weeks I had to have that terminated.

Fiona: So that was really the first sort of inkling that I had ... that there was something very bizarre and wrong with the way I was using drugs and drink, so I decided to go and live in Poland because that would then fix everything. So then I went to, to live in Poland where the vodka was cheap and all that sort of thing, ended up going to prison in Poland, for beating up an air hostess and a pilot on an aeroplane, came home from Poland in 1997 because by this stage work was beginning to affect my drinking. In Poland I took my first morning drink.

Aaron: So work started to affect your drinking?

Fiona: At this stage I was earning £120,000 a year, so I was still a high-achieving, functioning alcoholic, and I had enough money put by, to give up work, and I'd also been diagnosed with cancer, it's all quite convoluted, this story, ... so I'd had enough. I was earning all this money, that had been my dream, and I had my massive car, and I had my house and I had all this stuff, and none of it was making me feel anything other than just desperate.

Aaron: And how old were you at that point?

Fiona: 39. So I came back to England, and I'd been diagnosed with cancer and I thought, well, do you know what, I'm going to try and drink myself to death and if that doesn't work then the cancer will kill me. So that was in the September, 1997. By December – despite the drinking, I was still waking up every morning, and I wasn't dead, so I thought, do you know what, I might actually go and speak to somebody about this. I went to one of the local alcohol teams, and they said, well, look, we want you to keep this diary. Now at this point I knew I had a problem,

Aaron: So just to be clear – how did you know you had a problem?

Fiona: Because I'd made the decision that I was going to go home and drink myself to death. But I thought the drinking was just because of this terrible life that I'd had and God killed my baby, you know, there was no responsibility for me in, in all of this. So then they said, look, we'll try a home detox and we'll start you on January the 10th. And I thought, oh, I can't do that it's my 40th birthday on January the 11th. So I put them off doing that and I had this massive party, and I don't actually remember the next three weeks at all. And I came out of that and this was what took me in recovery, bearing in mind I'd basically murdered a baby, I'd been to prison, all sorts of other stuff had happened, but I woke up, probably about four o'clock one morning, thinking, I'm not going to have a drink today. And even as I was thinking it I was going down the stairs, and it was like I'd turned into two people. One that didn't want to drink and one that was going to do it. And I stood there and watched myself drink vodka from a bottle and thought, I can't do this any more. And that was it.

Aaron: Can you explain that?

Fiona: No. Absolutely not at all.

Aaron: That's very interesting, isn't it? So at some level you made a decision you don't want to do this and at another level, behaviour continues? And the two are kind of separate. Although from what you said before you'd had those kinds of similar experiences, perhaps not as stark, at an early age in terms of experiencing a kind of ambivalence? A kind of contradiction around your ... behaviour?

Fiona: I had been diagnosed with a dissociative identity disorder. That came when I was in, in recovery, and, yes, I could see that. That I'd been living sort of three different lives and I couldn't cross them, and that was a really hard part of, of my recovery, so by this stage then, yes, my mental health problems were really quite severe. So I paid for myself to go into a rehab, because I didn't know what else to do. Then that was it, the doctor said to me, Fiona, just don't drink. And I sat and I looked at him and I said, and how am I going to do that? So he wasn't willing to help but there again I'd not been very pleasant, because I'd been in the surgery several times under the influence, so there was quite a lot of ground to make up when I was trying to stop drinking.

Aaron: So you went into rehab? What sort of experience was that?

Fiona: Terrifying. Absolutely terrified.

Aaron: Did you stay the course?

Fiona: I stayed there six weeks, it was a four-week course, they asked me to stay another two weeks because they didn't think I was quite getting the hang of it, but I didn't, didn't drink, and also straight from there I went into hospital and had the cancer sorted out so the early recovery was really a bit bizarre, and I drank twice after that. On the first occasion I don't really know what happened but I was arrested from my garden shed, and almost sectioned. Then it was another three months after that I'd gone out working at my old job, and I was out in Estonia, and took cocaine and drank, ending up fighting on the tramlines with prostitutes, lost all my money, jewellery, and was almost deported. That was the last drink I ever took.

Aaron: Right. How long ago was that?

Fiona: October the 19th 1998.

Aaron: So you went into rehab first in March 98? So the last drink you had was October 98? So actually that was quite a rapid recovery in the scheme of things because you went into your first rehab ... and it clearly made an impact on you?

Fiona: I drank on July the 17th, and that's when I got arrested from my garden shed, that was about ... I, I remember at eight o'clock in the evening being sober and that was two o'clock the next morning that I was arrested from my garden shed, so probably eight hours of drinking, no more, and October the 19th was I set out on that evening again around about eight o'clock, and it was over by midnight.

(Continued)

(Continued)

Aaron: So was rehab essentially a twelve-step programme?

Fiona: Yes. But the important thing was actually the counsellor I had, I think, I was in counselling for, oh, God, two years, from the rehab.

Fiona: Yeah. And then I went from there, because I was also referred to the National Hospital for Neurology because they wanted, to put me on an experimental programme, for this dystonia and paralysis. But the counsellor in the rehab thought I had some deeper issues than he could deal with and so they ... the physical therapy was to treat it like a stroke and try and move the function around, but they insisted I had psychotherapy, at the same time, and that was with somebody who was a drug-addiction counsellor who was a specialist in dissociative identity disorder. Because they didn't think I'd be able to recover properly. Because part of the problem was it was brain damage that they think had been caused by my parents and they needed to make me face it full on. Before the therapy would work. If that makes any sense?

Aaron: It does, I mean, did it make sense to you?

Fiona: Oh yes, in the end, yeah.

Aaron: .... there's an argument, isn't there, that, in terms of looking at some of those deeper issues, whether in terms of overcoming your addition, whether you need to address those other issues.

Fiona: Yes.

Aaron: And it sounds like what you're saying is, for you this was important.

Fiona: Yes it was.

Aaron: So you've used and you continue to use AA? What are the benefits of that, of AA, would you argue?

Fiona: Like-minded people. For me, I'll tell you what the main benefit was is that because I started drinking so early I never really had a blueprint for a grown-up life at all, I'd never taken responsibility for myself. The twelve-step programme gave me a way of actually putting a life together. And allows me to, to live my life and deal with problems. When I was ten weeks sober my adoptive father died, because I was in AA I was looked after ... And six weeks later my adoptive mother died, that was followed by every single person in that adoptive family apart from my adoptive brother, died in the first six months. Interestingly I needed the support because I wasn't upset, I was happy. I was free at last and I didn't know what to do with that. And because it's such a caring community, I was looked after, I knew absolutely nobody when I got into recovery, I was completely on my own.

Aaron: So that's interesting, in terms of actually giving a framework for living are the spiritual dimensions important to that?

Fiona: Yes.

Aaron: As well, to you?

Fiona: Yeah.

Aaron: Is that as a Christian or as having an active faith, or ... ?

Fiona: I don't ... Well, I have no religion ... When I look back, between the ages of 11 to about 21 I was heavily into church, I was a Sunday School teacher, I was always searching for something, um, so I think this spiritual dimension where you can choose your own faith basically, was what I was looking for.

Aaron: Is there any sense in which AA has actually filled a kind of gap in your life?

Fiona: Yes.

Aaron: Or a void in your life. So it gives you your recovery ...

Fiona: Yes.

Aaron: So have you been involved in the same group all the way along, or ... ?

Fiona: No, I moved here five years ago now from St Albans, so I needed to move away from there because when I first got into recovery there I was paralysed down one side and all anybody ever remembers was this, this limping, shuffling person whose parents both died in the first four months, and it was like, oh, if Fiona can do it you can do it. And I'd always been really looked after, I needed to move away and start a new life and stand on my own two feet.

Aaron: So given your situation now, given that you're an academic ... with an interest in complexity theory ... lots of what you talked about just fits very nicely within that complexity paradigm. If you take a paradigm like complexity what are the benefits of using that in relation to addiction? What are the implications for their recovery?

Fiona: For me learning about this stuff, the, the holistic view, I know that at the end of my drinking I was tunnel-visioned and it's very difficult to get out of that when you've lived your life in, in that sort of way for so long, so it's sort of opened up my view, it's allowed me to get out of the debating society on what causes addiction, it's certainly done that because it really doesn't matter. I don't think it's one thing, I think it's a whole number of things. I believe that if I'd have been brought up in the most cosseted household there ever was I would have ended up being an alcoholic. However, I believe my behaviour wouldn't have been as destructive, it wouldn't have happened so early, and, and maybe the depth of it wouldn't have been so bad. So that's what I think. I also think alcohol helped me to survive those early years ...

Aaron: That's interesting. So you can use alcohol as a kind of coping mechanism?

Fiona: Yeah.

Aaron: So in the language of complexity you're using it in a particular way, but then the problem starts to take on a life of its own?

Fiona: Yes. The solution becomes the problem in place of the problem and starts to escalate. But this is the way it was for me, I would drink and cause an incident ... and therefore in order to get over the shame and guilt

(Continued)

(Continued)

of that incident I'd drink more. And another incident would happen that would be so much bigger that that incident would look quite small. And that became a way of life. When I went to prison this is me – earning 120 grand ... in a cell thinking, shit, how did this happen? But the dead baby all those weeks ago suddenly pales into insignificance, so I can get rid of that shame and guilt ... and this is all part of the complexity I think of, of the problem, because it becomes a way of life in dealing with it. And then because of all this guilt and shame you've got an excuse to drink.

Aaron: So you're, you're constantly acting to protect the drinking and the drinking behaviour is dynamic and informs everything else ... ?

Fiona: Yes ...

Conclusion

Complex intractable problems such as addiction are examples of what policy makers are calling 'Wicked problems', that is problems that cannot be solved simply by an improvement in each of the agencies involved (Bovaird and Loffler, 2003). In essence this means that a whole systems approach is required that does not simply seek to break down the problem into its component parts, with differing agencies dealing with each one. It is evident from the research covered in this book that a multi-modal approach is required to address complex issues such as an addiction to psychoactive substances and the harms that it causes. Within the context of case management there may be a range of organisations from prescribing services, to housing providers, to counsellors involved in any one case. However, as has been demonstrated it is the human relationship which is central to effective working and is seen to be essential to the service user. Complexity theory shows us that any intervention within a system will have intended and unintended consequences; it may be, for example, that one of the reasons that coerced interventions amplify and distort outcomes from service delivery is precisely because a genuine positive regard for an individual and punishment are not compatible bedfellows. Broadly speaking, a move towards care management and integrated care pathways and a concern for the patients' journey recognise the importance of a whole system approach but have failed to address the issue of the human relationship within what can become a bureaucratic nightmare for worker and service user alike (see Pycroft and Gough, 2010).

In searching for higher order solutions to complex problems then Orford (2008) has argued that rigorous psychosocial interventions such CBT, or MET, or TSF are all essentially doing the same thing. Research into effective working with substance misusers continues to demonstrate the importance of sensitivity and the application of motivational skills. These skills are acquired by workers in their broad everyday lives and are specific to working in a professionalised environment; it is developed less by formal training than by an interaction with clients combined with individualised feedback from expert coaches (Ashton, 2009).

It is this way of relating as human beings, and the values that it encompasses, that needs to be explored as well as developed further information of effective interventions. If we found ourselves experiencing problems with psychoactive substances then we would expect nothing less than kindness, compassion, and empathy.

Bibliography

Advisory Council on the Misuse of Drugs (ACMD) (2006) *Pathways to Problems: Hazardous Use of Tobacco, Alcohol and Other Drugs by Young People in the UK and Its Implications for Policy*. London: Advisory Council on the Misuse of Drugs.

Anglin, D., Connor, M., Bradley, T., Annon, J. and Longshore, D. (2007) 'Levo-alpha-acetyl-methadol versus methadone maintenance: 1 year treatment retention, outcomes and status', *Addiction, 102*, 1432–42.

Alcoholics Anonymous (2008) www.alcoholicsanonymous.org/en_services_for_members.cfm?PageID=98&SubPage=117. Retrieved 13 March 2008.

Ashton, M. (1999) 'Project MATCH: unseen colossus', *Drug and Alcohol Findings, 1*(1).

Ashton, M. (2009) *The Motivational Hallo, Manners Matter*. London: Drugscope.

Babor, T. (1992) 'Substance-related problems in the context of international classificatory systems'. In M. Lader, G. Edwards and D.C. Drummond (eds), *The Nature of Alcohol and Drug Related Problems*. Oxford: Oxford Medical Publications.

Babor, T., Caetano, R., Casswell, S., Edwards, G., Giesbrecht, N., Graham, Kathryn, Grube, J., Gruenewald, P., Hill, L., Holder, H., Homel, R., Osterberg, E., Rehm, R., Room, R. and Rossow, I. (2003) *Alcohol: No Ordinary Commodity, Research and Public Policy*. Oxford: Oxford University Press.

Ball, A.L. (2007) 'HIV, injecting drug use and harm reduction: a public health response', *Addiction, 102*, 684–90.

Ball, D., Pembrey, M. and Stephens, D. (2007) 'Genomics'. In D. Nutt, T. Robbins, G. Stimson, M. Ince and A. Jackson (eds), *Drugs and the Future*. London: Elsevier. pp. 89–132.

Bandura, A. (1977) 'Self efficacy: toward a unifying theory of behavioral change', *Psychological Review, 84*, 191–215.

Barber, J. (1995) *Social Work with Addiction*. Basingstoke: Macmillan.

Barkow, J., Cosmides, L. and Tooby, J. (1992) *The Adapted Mind: Evolutionary Psychology and the Generation of Culture*. Oxford: Oxford University Press.

Barnard, M.A. and McKeganey, N.P. (2004) 'The impact of parental problem drug use on children: what is the problem and what is being done to help?', *Addiction, 99*(5): 552–559.

Bar-Yam, Y. (1997) *Dynamics of Complex Systems*. Cambridge, MA: Perseus.

Baugh, J. (1988) 'Gaining control by giving strategies for coping with powerlessness'. In W.A. Miller and J.E. Martin (eds), *Behavior Therapy and Religion Integrating Spiritual and Behavioral Approaches to Change*. Newbury Park, CA: Sage.

Beckett, H., Heap, J., McArdle, P., Gilvarry, E., Christian, J., Bloor, R., Crome, I. and Frischer, M. (2004) *Understanding Problem Drug Use Among Young People Accessing*

Drug Services: A Multivariate Approach Using Statistical Modelling Techniques. London: Home Office.

Bentley, D. (2004) 'Genomes for medicine', *Nature, 429*(27 May).

Berridge, V. (2002) 'Epidemiology and policy: the post-war context', *Bulletin on Narcotics, 1 and 2.*

Berridge,V. (2005) 'The "British System" and its history: myth and reality'. In J. Strang and M. Gossop (eds), *Heroin Addiction and the British System: Volume One Origins and Evolution.* London: Routledge.

Bickel, W. and Potenza, M. (2006) 'The forest and the trees: addiction as a complex self-organizing system'. In W. Miller and K. Carroll (eds), *Rethinking Substance Abuse: What the Science Shows and What We Should Do About It.* New York: Guilford Press. pp. 8–21.

Bilton, T.,Bonnett, K.,Jones, P.,Lawson,T., Skinner, D., Stanworth, M., and Webster, A. (2002) *Introductory Sociology,* (4th edition). Basingstoke. Palgrave Macmillan.

Bovaird, T. and Loffer, E. (2003) 'Evaluating the quality of public governance: indicators, models and methodologies', *International Review of Administrative Sciences, 69,* 313–28.

Braithwaite, J., Iedema, R.A. and Jorm, C. (2007) 'Trust, communication, theory of mind and social brain hypothesis: deep explanations for what goes wrong in health care', *Journal of Health Organisation and Management, 21*(4–5), 353–67.

Breakwell, G. and Rowett, C. (1982) *Social Work: The Social Psychological Approach.* Netherlands:Van Nostran Reinhold Company.

Brugal, M., Domingo-Salvany, A., Puig, R., Barrio, G., Garcia de Olalla, P. and de la Fuente, L. (2005) 'Evaluating the impact of methadone maintenance programmes on mortality due to overdose and aids in a cohort of heroin users in Spain', *Addiction, 100*(7), 981–9.

Buchman,T. (2002) 'The community of the self', *Nature,* November.

Buckland, P. (2008) 'Will we ever find the genes for addiction?', *Addiction, 103.*

Cabinet Office (2004) *Alcohol Harm Reduction Strategy for England.* London. Strategy Unit.

Caulkins, J.P. ((2007)) 'The need for dynamic drug policy', *Addiction, 102,* 4–7.

Chick, J. (2002) 'Evolutionary psychobiology: any relevance for therapy?', *Addiction,* 97(4), 473–4.

Cook, C. (2004) 'Addiction and spirituality', *Addiction, 99,* 539–51.

Cooper, H., Braye, S. and Geyer, R. (2008) 'Complexity and interprofessional education', *Learning in Health and Social Care, 3*(4), 179–89.

Curran, V. and Drummond, C. (2007) 'Psychological treatments of substance misuse and dependence'. In D. Nutt, T. Robbins, G. Stimson, M. Ince and A. Jackson (eds), *Drugs and the Future: Brain Science, Addiction and Society.* London: Academic Press.

Dackis, C. and O' Brien, C. (2005) 'Neurobiology of addiction: treatment and public policy ramifications', *Nature Neuroscience 8,* 1431–6.

Darke, S., Degenhardt, L. and Mattick, R. (2007) *Mortality Amongst Illicit Drug Users: Epidemiology, Causes and Intervention.* Cambridge: Cambridge University Press.

Darke, S. (2008) 'Truth is not always found in the laboratory', *Addiction, 103,* 1063–8.

Davenport-Hines, R. (2001) *The Pursuit of Oblivion: A Global History of Narcotics, 1500–2000.* London:Weidenfeld and Nicolson.

Davenport-Hines, R. (2004) *The Pursuit of Oblivion: A Social History of Drugs*. London: Phoenix.

Davoli, M., Bargagli, A.M., Perucci, C.A., Schifano, P., Belleudi, V., Hickman, M., Salamina, G., Diecedue, R., Vigna-Taglianti, F. and Faggiano, F. (2007) 'Risk of fatal overdose during and after specialist drug treatment: the VEdeTTE study, a national multi-site prospective cohort study', *Addiction, 102*, 1954–9.

Dawkins, R. (2006) *The Selfish Gene* (30th anniversary edition). Oxford: Oxford University Press.

Department of Health (1999) *Drug Misuse and Dependence – Guidelines on Clinical Management*. London: Department of Health.

Department of Health (2004) *Alcohol Needs Assessment Research Project*. London: Department of Health.

DiClemente, C. and Prochaska, J. (1998) 'Toward a comprehensive, transtheoretical model of change, stages of change and addictive behaviour'. In W. Miller and N. Heather (eds), *Treating Addictive Behaviours* (2nd edition). New York: Plenum. pp. 3–24.

Drake, R., Essock, S., Shaner, A., Carey, K., Minkoff, K., Kola, L., Lyne, D., Osher, F., Clarke, R. and Rickards, L. (2004) 'Implementing dual diagnosis services for clients with severe mental illness', *Journal of Life Long Learning in Psychiatry, 11*(1), 102–10.

Drucker, E., Lurie, P., Wodak, A. and Alcabes, P. (1998) 'Measuring harm reduction: the effects of needle and syringe exchange programmes and methadone maintenance on the ecology of HIV', *AIDS. 12 (suppl A)*, 217–30.

Drummond, D. Collin (1992) 'Problems and dependence: chalk and cheese or bread and butter?' In M. Lader, G. Edwards and D.C. Drummond (eds), *The Nature of Alcohol and Drug Related Problems*. Oxford: Oxford University Press.

Dudley, R. (2000) 'Evolutionary origins of human alcoholism in primate frugivory', *The Quarterly Review of Biology, 75*(1).

Dudley, R. (2002) 'Fermenting fruit and the historical ecology of ethanol ingestion: is alcoholism in modern humans an evolutionary hangover', *Addiction, 97*.

Duke, K. (2003) *Drugs, Prisons and Policy-Making*. Basingstoke: Palgrave-Macmillan.

Dweck, C. (2000) *Self-Theories: Their Role in Motivation, Personality and Development*. Philadelphia: Psychology Press: Taylor Francis Group.

Edwards, G., Anderson, P., Babor, T., Caswell, S., Ferrence, R., Giesbrecht, N., Godfrey, C., Holder, H., Lemmens, P., Makela, K., Midanik, L., Norstrom, R., Osterberg, E., Romelsjo, A., Room, R., Simpura, J. and Skog, O. (1994) *Alcohol Policy and the Public Good*. Oxford: Oxford University Press.

Edwards, G. (2004) *Matters of Substance: Drugs, Is Legalization the Right Answer – Or the Wrong Question?* London: Penguin Books.

Edwards, G. (2007) 'How the 1977 World Health Organisation report on alcohol-related disabilities came to be written: a provisional analysis', *Addiction, 102*(11), 1711–21.

Edwards, G., Anderson, P., Babor, T., Casswell, S., Ferrence, R., Giesbrecht, N., Godfrey, C., Holder, H., Lemmens, P., Makela, K., Midanik, L., Norstrom, T., Osterberg, E., Romelsjo, A., Room, R., Simpura, J. and Skog, O. (1995). *Alcohol Policy and the Public Good*. Oxford: Oxford University Press.

Edwards, G. and Gross, M. (1976) 'Alcohol dependence: provisional description of a clinical syndrome', *British Medical Journal*, 1058–61.

Emler, N. (2001) *Self-Esteem: The Costs and Causes of Low Self Worth*. York: Joseph Rowntree Foundation.

European Monitoring Centre for Drugs and Drug Addiction (EMCDDA) (2006, 05/10/09) Annual Report.

Eysenck, M. (1993) *Principles of Cognitive Psychology*. Hove: Taylor and Francis.

Farrell, M. and Raistrick, D. (2005) 'Oral methadone maintenance programmes'. In J. Strang and M. Gossop (eds), *Heroin Addiction and the British System*. Abingdon: Routledge. pp. 105–20.

Fazey, C. (2003) 'The Commission on Narcotic Drugs and the United Nations International Drug Control Programme: politics, policies and prospect for change', *The International Journal of Drug Policy, 14*(2), 155–69.

Fiorentine, R. (1998) 'Effective drug treatment: testing the distal needs hypothesis', *Journal of Substance Abuse Treatment, 15*(4), 281–9.

Fleming, P. (2005) 'Experimental amphetamine maintenance prescribing'. In J. Strang and M. Gossop (eds), *Heroin Addiction and the British System Volume 2*. Abingdon: Routledge. pp. 131–44.

Forrester, D., Pokhrel, S., McDonald, L., Copello, A., Binne, C., Jensch, G., Wasbein, C. and Giannou, D. (2008) *Final Report on the Evaluation of 'Option 2'*. Cardiff: Welsh Assembly Government.

Frith, C.D. (2004) 'Schizophrenia and Theory of Mind', *Psychological Medicine, 34*, 385–9.

Fry, C., Koshnood, K., Power, R. and Sharma, M. (2008) 'Harm reduction ethics: acknowledging the values and beliefs behind our actions', *International Journal of Drug Policy, 19*(1), 1–3.

Gardner, D. (2009) *Risk: The Science and Politics of Fear*. London: Virgin Books.

Gateley, I. (2001) *La Diva Nicotina*. London: Simon and Schuster.

Gerald, M. and Higley, J. (2002) 'Evolutionary underpinnings of excessive alcohol consumption', *Addiction, 97*.

Giesbrecht, N. (2007) 'Reducing alcohol related damage in populations: rethinking the roles of education and persuasion interventions', *Addiction, 102*, 1345–9.

Gifford, E. and Humphreys, K. (2007) 'The psychological science of addiction', *Addiction, 102*, 352–61.

Goldstein, A. (2001) *Addiction: From Biology to Drug Policy*. Oxford: Oxford University Press.

Gossop, M., Marsden, J., Stewart, P., Lehmann, C., Edwards, C., Wilson, A. and Segar, G. (1998) 'Substance use, health and social problems of service users at 54 drug treatment agencies: intake data from the National Outcome Research Study', *British Journal of Psychiatry, 173*, 166–71.

Gossop, M. (2000) *Living With Drugs*. Aldershot: Ashgate.

Gossop, M., Marsden, J., Stewart, D. and Kidd, T. (2003) 'The National Treatment Outcome Research Study (NTORS): 4–5 year follow-up results', *Addiction, 98*(3), 291–303.

Gossop, M., Neto, D., Radovanovic, M., Batra, A., Toteva, S., Musalek, M., Skutle, A. and Goos, C. (2007) 'Physical health problems among patients seeking treatment for alcohol use disorders: a study in six European cities', *Addiction Biology, 12*(2), 190–6.

Graves, R. (1992) *The Greek Myths*. London: Penguin.

Guastello, S.J. and Liebovitch, L. (2009) 'Introduction to nonlinear dynamics and complexity. In S.J. Guastello, M. Koopmans and D. Pincus (eds), *Chaos and Complexity in Psychology: The Theory of Nonlinear Dynamical Systems*. Cambridge: Cambridge University Press. pp. 1–36.

Hall, W., Carter, K. and Morley, K. (2003) 'Addiction, neuroscience and ethics', *Addiction, 98*(7), 867–70.

Hall, W. (2006) 'Avoiding potential misuses of addiction brain science', *Addiction, 101*, 1529–32.

Healthcare Commission and National Treatment Agency for Substance Misuse (2008) *Improving Services for Substance Misuse*. London: Healthcare Commission.

Heather, N. and Robertson, I. (1981) *Controlled Drinking*. London: Methuen.

Heather, N. and Robertson, I. (1997) *Problem Drinking* (3rd edition). Oxford: Oxford University Press.

Hesselbrock, V. and Hesselbrock, M. (2006) 'Developmental perspectives on the risk for developing substance abuse problems. In W. Miller and K. Carroll (eds), *Rethinking Substance Abuse: What the Science Shows and What We Should Do About It*. New York: Guilford Press.

Hickman, M., Madden, P., Henry, J., Baker, A., Wallace, C., Wakefield, J., Stimson, G. and Elliott (2003) 'Trends in drug overdose deaths in England and Wales 1993–1998: methadone does not kill more people than heroin', *Addiction, 98*, 419–25.

Hickman, M., Vickerman, P., Macleod, J., Kirkbride, J. and Jone, P. (2007) 'Cannabis and schizophrenia: model projections of the impact of the rise in cannabis use on historical and future trends in schizophrenia in England and Wales', *Addiction, 102*(4), 597–606.

Hickman, M., Lingford-Hughes, A., Bailey, C., Macleod, J., Nut, D. and Henderson, G. (2008) 'Does alcohol increase the risk of overdose death: the need for a translational approach', *Addiction, 103*, 1060–2.

Hill, E. and Newlin, D. (2002) 'Evolutionary approaches to addiction: an introduction', *Addiction, 97*(4): 375–9.

HM Government (1995) *Tackling Drugs Together*. London: HMSO.

Holder, H. (1999) *Alcohol and the Community: A Systems Approach to Prevention*. Cambridge: Cambridge University Press.

Holt, T. (2004) 'Introduction'. In T. Holt (ed.), *Complexity for Clinicians*. Oxford: Radcliffe. pp. 3–13.

Home Office (1998) *Tackling Drugs to Build a Better Britain*. London: Home Office.

Home Office (2000) *British Crime Survey and Other Surveys*. London: Home Office.

Home Office (2002) *Updated Drug Strategy*. London: Home Office.

Home Office (2004) *Alcohol Harm Reduction Strategy for England and Wales*. London: Home Office.

Home Office (2007) *Offender Management Caseload Statistics*. London: Home Office.

Home Office (2008). *Drugs: Protecting Families and Communities, the 2008 Drug Strategy*. London: Home Office.

House of Commons Science and Technology Committee (2005/2006) *Drugs Classification: Making a Hash of It?* London: House of Commons.

Hughes, J. (2007) 'Defining dependence: describing symptom clusters versus central constructs', *Addiction, 102*(11), 1531–8.

Humphreys, K. (2004) *Circles of Recovery: Self Help Organisations for Addictions.* Cambridge: Cambridge University Press.

Humphreys, K. and Gifford, E. (2006) 'Religion, spirituality, and the troublesome use of substances'. In W. Miller and K. Carroll (eds), *Rethinking Substance Abuse: What the Science Shows and What We Should Do About It.* New York: Guilford Press. pp. 257–74.

Humphreys, K. and Tucker, J.A. (2002) 'Toward more responsive and effective intervention systems for alcohol-related problems', *Addiction, 97*(2), 126–132.

Hunt, G. (2007) "Combining different substances in the dance scene; enhancing pleasure and managing risk." Unpublished conference presentation at the British Society of Criminology Annual Conference at the London School of Economics 19th September

Hyman, S. and Malenka, R. (2001) 'Addiction and the brain: the neurobiology of compulsion and its persistence'. *Nature Reviews Neuroscience, 2,* 695–703.

Imel, Z.E. and Wampold, B.E. (2008) 'Distinctions without a difference: direct comparisons of psychotherapies for alcohol use disorders', *Psychology of Addictive Behaviors, 22*(4), 533–43.

Institute of Medicine (1990) *Broadening the Base for the Treatment of Alcohol Problems.* Washington, DC: National Academy Press.

Koob, G. (2006) 'The neurobiology of addiction: a hedonic Calvinist view', In W. Miller and K. Carroll (eds), *Rethinking Substance Abuse: What the Science Shows and What We Should Do About It.* New York: Guilford Press. pp. 25–45.

Jones, A.,Weston, S.,Moody, A., Millar, T.,Dollin, L., Anderson, T. and Donmall, M. (2007) *The drug treatment outcomes research study (DTORS)baseline report.* London. Home Office.

Koob, G. and Le Moal, M. (2001) 'Drug addiction, dysregulation of reward, and allostasi', *Neuropsychopharmacology, 24*(2), 97–129.

Lader, M., Edwards, G. and Drummond, D.C. (eds) (1992) *The Nature of Alcohol and Drug Related Problems.* Oxford: Oxford University Press.

Lende, D. and Smith, E. (2002) 'Evolution meets biopsychosociality: an analysis of addictive behaviour', *Addiction, 97*(4): 447–58.

Leshner, A. (2007) 'Addiction is a brain disease'. *Issues in Science and Technology.* www.issues.org/17.3/leshner.htm Retrieved 15 October 2009.

Levine, H. (2003) 'Global drug prohibition its uses and crises', *International Journal of Drug Policy, 14,* 145–53.

Li, T.K., Brenda, D. and Grant, B.F. (2007a) 'The Alcohol Dependence Syndrome: 30 years later: a commentary', *Addiction, 102*(10), 1522–30.

Li, T.K., Brenda, D. and Grant, B.F. (2007b) 'The Alcohol Dependence Syndrome, 30 years later – a response to the commentaries', *Addiction, 102*(10), 1531–8.

Liappas, J., Lascaratos, J., Fouti, S. and Christodoulou, G. (2003) 'Alexander the Great's relationship with alcohol', *Addiction, 98,* 561–7.

Lindstrom, L. (1992) *Managing Alcoholism: Matching Clients to Treatments.* Oxford: Oxford Medical Publications.

Lintzeris, N., Strang, J., Metrebian, N., Byford, S., Hallam, C., Lee, S., Zador, D. and RIOTT Group (2006) 'Methodology for the Randomised Injecting Opioid Treatment Trial (RIOTT): evaluating injectable methadone and injectable heroin treatment versus optimised oral methadone treatment in the UK', *Journal of Harm Reduction, 3(28)*.

Longshore, D., Annon, J., Anglin, M. Douglas, M., Rawson and Richard, A. (2005) 'Levo-alpha-acetyl-methadol versus methadone: treatment retention and opiate use', *Addiction, 100(8)*, 1131–9.

Marlatt, G.A. and Gordon, J.R. (eds) (1985) *Relapse Prevention: Maintenance Strategies in the Treatment of Addictive Behaviors*. New York: Guilford Press.

Marlatt, G.A., Baer, J. and Quigley, L. (1995) 'Self-efficacy and addictive behavior' In A. Bandura (ed.), *Self Efficacy in Changing Societies*. Cambridge: Cambridge University Press. pp. 289–315.

Marsden, J., Boys, A., Farrell, M., Stillwell, G., Hutchings, K., Hillebrand, J. et al. (2005) 'Personal and social correlates of alcohol consumption among mid-adolescents', *British Journal of Developmental Psychology, 23*, 427–50.

Martinson, R. (1974) 'What works? Questions and answers about prison reform', *Public Interest, 35*, 22–54.

Maruna, S. (2001) *Making Good: How Ex Convicts Reform and Rebuild Their Lives*. Washington, DC: American Psychological Association.

Maruna, S. and Immarigeon, R. (2004) *After Crime and Punishment: Pathways to Offender Reintegration*. Cullompton: Willan.

McGuire, J. (ed.) (1995) *What Works: Reducing Re-offending, Guidelines from Research and Practice*. Chichester: Wiley.

McKay, J. and McLellan, A. (1998) 'Deciding where to start: working with polyproblem individuals'. In W. Miller and N. Heather (eds), *Treating Addictive Behaviors*. New York: Plenum. pp. 173–86.

McLellan, T. (2002) 'Have we evaluated addiction treatment correctly? Implications from a chronic care perspective', *Addiction, 97(3)*, 249–52.

McLellan, T., McKay, J., Forman, R., Cacciola, J. and Kemp, J. (2005) 'Reconsidering the evaluation of addiction treatment from retrospective follow up to concurrent recovery monitoring', *Addiction, 100(4)*, 447–58.

McLellan, T. (2006) 'What we need is a system: creating a responsive and effective substance abuse treatment system'. In W. Miller and K. Carroll (eds), *Rethinking Substance Abuse: What the Science Shows and What We Should Do About It*. New York: Guilford Press. pp. 275–92.

McSweeney, T., Stevens, N., Hunt, A. and Turnbull, P. (2006) 'Twisting arms or a helping hand? Assessing the impact of coerced and comparable voluntary drug treatment options', *The British Journal of Criminology, 47(3)*, 470–91.

McSweeney, T. and Hough, M. (2006) 'Supporting offenders with multiple needs: lessons for the "mixed economy" model of service provision', *Criminology and Criminal Justice, 6(1)*, 107–25.

Means, R., Richards, S. and Smith, R. (2003) *Community Care: Policy and Practice*. Basingstoke: Palgrave Macmillan.

Measham, F. (2006) 'The new policy mix: alcohol, harm minimisation, and determined drunkenness in contemporary society', *International Journal of Drug Policy, 17(4)*, 258–68.

Meltzer, H. (1995) *OPCS Surveys of Psychiatric Morbidity in Great Britain: Report 1: The Prevalence of Psychiatric Morbidity among Adults Living in Private Households*. London: Office of Population Census and Surveys.

Miller, W. (2006) 'Motivational factors in addictive behaviors'. In W. Miller and K. Carroll (eds), *Rethinking Substance Abuse: What the Science Shows and What We Should Do About It*. New York: Guilford Press. pp. 134–50.

Miller, W. and Rollnick, S. (2002) *Motivational Interviewing: Preparing People for Change*. New York: Guilford Press.

Miller, W., Andrews, N., Wilbourne, P. and Bennet, M. (1998) 'A wealth of alternatives: effective treatments for alcohol problems'. In W. Miller and N. Heather (ed.), *Treating Addictive Behaviors* (2nd edition). New York: Plenum.

Moore, D. (2005) 'Key moments in the ethnography of drug related harm: reality checks for policy makers'. In T. Stockwell, P.J. Gruenewald, J.W.J. Toumbourou and W. Loxley (eds), *Preventing Harmful Substance Use: The Evidence Base for Policy and Practice*. Chichester: Wiley. pp. 433–42.

Morgan, M., Hibell, B., Andersson, B., Bjarnason, T., Kokkevi, A. and Narusk, A. (1999) 'The ESPAD study: implications for prevention', *Drugs – Education Prevention and Policy, 6*(2), 243–56.

Mruk, C. (1999) *Self-Esteem, Research, Theory and Practice*. Basingstoke: Free Association Books.

Mueser, K., Drake, R. and Wallach, M. (1998) 'Dual diagnosis: a review of aetiological theories', *Addictive Behaviors, 23*(6), 717–34.

National Treatment Agency for Substance Misuse (2001) *Models of Care for Adult Drug Users*. London: National Treatment Agency.

National Treatment Agency for Substance Misuse (2004) *Mapping of Department of Health's Standards for Better Health against Standards for the Substance Misuse Field*. London: National Treatment Agency.

National Treatment Agency for Substance Misuse (2005) *Nurse Prescribing in Substance Misuse*. London: National Treatment Agency.

National Treatment Agency for Substance Misuse (2006) *Models of Care for Treatment of Adult Drug Users, Update*. London: National Treatment Agency.

National Treatment Agency for Substance Misuse (2007) *The NTA's 2006 National Prescribing Audit: An Assessment of Prescribing Practices for Opioid Substitution Treatment in England 2004–05*. London: National Treatment Agency.

National Treatment Agency for Substance Misuse (2008) www.nta.nhs.uk/about_treatment/Types_of_treatment.aspx Retrieved 19 May 2008.

National Treatment Agency for Substance Misuse (2008) 'Types of treatment'. www.nta.nhs.uk/about_treatment/Types_of_treatment.aspx Retrieved 15 October 2009.

National Treatment Agency for Substance Misuse/Department of Health (2008) *Reducing Drug Related Harm: an Action Plan*. London: Department of Health.

National Treatment Agency for Substance Misuse (nd) *Commissioning Services to Reduce Drug Related Deaths*. London: National Treatment Agency.

Nesse, R. (2002) 'Evolution and addiction', *Addiction, 97*(4), 470–1.

Nestler, E. and Landsman, D. (February 2001) 'Learning about addiction from the genome', *Nature, 409*: 834–5.

Newburn, T. (2007) *Criminology*. Cullompton: Willan.

Newlin, D. (2002) 'The self-perceived survival ability and reproductive fitness (SPFit) theory of substance use disorders', *Addiction*, 97(4): 427 – 445.

Noble, D. (2006) *The Music of Life*. Oxford: Oxford University Press.

Office of the Deputy Prime Minister (2005) *Housing Support Options for Offenders who Misuse Substances*. London: ODPM.

Orford, J. (1990) 'Looking for synthesis in studying the nature of dependence: facing up to complexity'. In G. Edwards and M. Lader (eds), *The Nature of Drug Dependence*. Oxford: Oxford University Press. pp. 41–62.

Orford, J. (2002) *Excessive Appetites: A Psychological View of Addictions* (2nd edition). Chichester: Wiley.

Orford, J. (2008) 'Asking the right questions in the right way: the need for a shift in research on psychological treatments for addiction', *Addiction*, 103, 875–85.

Parker, H. (2005). 'Heroin epidemics and social exclusion in the UK 1980-2000', in J. Strang and M. Gossop (eds) *Heroin Addiction and the British System Vol 1*. London: Routledge.

Parker, H. Measham, F. and Aldridge, J. (1998) *Starting, Slowing, Switching and Stopping. Young People's Drug Pathways*. London: Home Office.

Partners, K.H. (2009) 'Untreatable or just hard to treat?' www.kingshealthpartners.org/khp/2009/09/15/untreatable-or-just-hard-to-treat/ Retrieved 14 October 2009.

Partridge, S. (2004) *Examining Case Management Models for Community Sentences*. London. Home Office.

Pawson, R. (2006) *Evidence-based Policy: A Realist Perspective*. London: SAGE.

Pawson, R. and Tilley, N. (1997) *Realistic Evaluation*. London: SAGE.

Pincus, D. (2009) 'Coherence, complexity and information flow: self-organizing processes in psychotherapy'. In S.J. Guastello, M. Koopmans and D. Pincus (eds), *Chaos and Complexity in Psychology: The Theory of Nonlinear Dynamical Systems*. Cambridge: Cambridge University Press. pp. 335–69.

Piper, T., Rudenstine, S., Stancliffe, S., Sherman, S., Nandi, V., Clear, A. et al. (2007) 'Overdose prevention for injecting drug users: lessons learned from Naloxone training and distribution programmes in New York City', *Harm Reduction Journal*, 25(4).

Pleace, N. (2008) *Effective Services for Substance Misuse and Homelessness in Scotland: Evidence from an International Review*. Edinburgh: Department for Communities and Local Government.

Plsek, P. and Greenhalgh, T. (2001) 'The challenge of complexity in health care', *British Medical Journal*, 323, 625–8.

Prochaska, J. and DiClemente, C. (1982) 'Transtheoretical therapy: towards a more integrative model of change', *Psychotherapy: Theory, Research and Practice*, 19, 276–8.

Project MATCH Research Group (1997) 'Matching alcoholism treatments to client heterogeneity: Project MATCH post treatment drinking outcomes', *Journal of Studies on Alcohol*, 58, 7–29.

Project MATCH (2005) http://www.commed.uchc.edu/match/ Accessed 11th January 2010

Pycroft, A. (2005) 'A new chance for rehabilitation: multi agency provision and potential under NOMS'. In J. Winstone and F. Pakes (eds), *Community Justice: Issues for Probation and Criminal Justice*. Cullompton: Willan. pp. 130–41.

Pycroft, A. and Gough, D. (eds) (2010) *Multi-Agency Working: Control and Care in Contemporary Correctional Practice*. Bristol: Policy Press.

Quirk, A., Lilly, R., Rhodes, T. and Stimson, G. (2003) 'Negotiating a script: the dynamics of staff/client relationships'. In G. Tober and J. Strang (eds), *Methadone Matters*. London: Martin Durnitz. pp. 38–44.

Raistrick, D., Heather, N. and Godfrey, C. (2006) *Review of the Effectiveness of Treatment for Alcohol Problems*. London: National Treatment Agency for Substance Misuse.

Ranganathan, S. (2005) *Relapse Management*. Chennai: United Nations Office of Drugs and Crime.

Ratcliffe, M. and Hutto, D. (2007) 'Introduction'. In D. Hutto, and M. Ratcliffe (eds), *Folk Psychology Re-assessed*. Dordrecht: Springer. pp. 1–24.

Regier, D., Farmer, M., Rae, D., Locke, B., Keith, S., Judd, L. and Goodwin, F. (1990) 'Comorbidity of mental disorders with alcohol and other drug abuse: results from the epidemiological catchment area (ECA) study', *Journal of the American Medical Association, 264,* 2511–18.

Rehm, J., Rehn, N., Room, R., Monteiro, M., Gmel, G., Jernigan, D. and Frick, U. (2003) 'The global distribution of average volume of alcohol consumption and patterns of drinking', *European Addiction Research, 9*(4).

Rehm, J.R.R., Graham, K., Monteiro, M., Gmel, G. and Sempos, C.T. (2003) 'The relationship of average volume of alcohol consumption and patterns of drinking to burden of disease: an overview', *Addiction, 98,* 1209–28.

Reuter, P. and Stevens, A. (2008) 'Assessing UK drug policy from a crime control perspective', *Criminology and Criminal Justice, 8*(4), 461–82.

Richards, D. and Smith, M. (2002) *Governance and Public Policy in the UK*. Oxford: Oxford University Press.

Robbins, T., Cardinal, R., DiCiano, P., Halligan, P., Hellemans, K., Lee, J. and Everitt, B. (2007) 'Neuroscience of drugs and addiction'. In D. Nutt, T. Robbins, G. Stimson, M. Ince and A. Jackson (eds), *Drugs and the Future*. London: Elsevier. pp. 11–88.

Roberts, M. and Eldridge, A. (2007) *Expecting 'Great Things?' The Impact of the Licensing Act 2002 on Democratic Involvement, Dispersal and Drinking Cultures*. London: Institute of Alcohol Studies.

Robson, G. and Marlatt, G.A. (2006) 'Harm reduction and alcohol policy', *International Journal of Drug Policy, 17,* 255–7.

Roffman, R. and Stephens, R. (eds) (2006) *Cannabis Dependence, its Nature, Consequences and Treatment*. Cambridge: Cambridge University Press.

Rosenberg, H., Melville, J. and McLean, P.C. (2002) 'Acceptability and availability of pharmacological interventions for substance misuse by British NHS treatment services'. *Addiction, 97,* 59–65.

Runciman. (1999) *Drugs and the Law: Report of the Independent Inquiry into the Misuse of Drugs Act 1971*. London: Police Foundation.

Russell, M. and Carruthers, S. (2005) 'The evidence base for preventing the spread of blood-borne diseases within and from populations of injecting drug users'. In T. Stockwell, P.J. Gruenewald, J.W. Toumbourou and W. Loxley (eds), *Preventing Harmful Substance Use: The Evidence Base for Policy and Practice*. Chichester: Wiley. pp. 367–80.

Saxe, R. and Baron-Cohen, S. (2006) 'Editorial: the neuroscience of theory of mind', *Social Neuroscience, 1*(3–4), i–ix.

Scottish Government. (2008) *The Road to Recovery: A New Approach to Tackling Scotland's Drug Problem*. Edinburgh: The Scottish Government.

Sebag-Montefiore, S. (2002) *Stalin: The Court of the Red Tsar*. London: Weidenfeld and Nicolson.

Seddon, R., Ralphs, R. and Williams, L. (2008) 'Risk, security and the criminalization of British drug policy', *British Journal of Criminology, 48*(6), 818–35.

Seddon, T. (2007) 'Coerced drug treatment in the criminal justice system: conceptual, ethical and criminological issues', *Criminology and Criminal Justice, 7*(3), 269–86.

Select Committee on Home Affairs (2002) Third Report THE GOVERNMENT'S DRUGS POLICY: IS IT WORKING? London: HMSO.

Senbanjo, R., Wolff, K. and Marshall, J. (2006) 'Excessive alcohol consumption is associated with reduced quality of life among methadone patients', *Addiction, 102*, 257–63.

Seymour, A., Black, M., Jay, J., Cooper, G., Weir, C. and Oliver, J. (2003) 'The role of methadone in drug-related deaths in the west of Scotland', *Addiction, 98*, 995–1002.

Sheehan, M. and Ridge, D. (2001) '"You become really close…you talk about the silly things you did, and we laugh": the role of binge drinking in female secondary students' lives', *Substance Use & Misuse, 36*(3), 347–72.

Sheldon, T. (2008) 'More than a quick fix', *British Medical Journal, 336*, 68–9.

Sheridan, J. (2005) 'Needle exchange in Britain'. In J. Strang and M. Gossop (eds), *Heroin Addiction and the British System*. Oxford: Routledge.

Social Exclusion Unit (2002) *Reducing Re-offending by Ex-prisoners*. London: HMSO.

Solberg, U., Burkhart, G. and Nilson, M. (2002) 'An overview of opiate substitution treatment in the European Union and Norway', *International Journal of Drug Policy, 13*(6): 477–484.

Stark, C., Kidd, B. and Sykes, R. (eds) (1999) *Illegal Drug Use in the United Kingdom: Prevention, Treatment and Enforcement*. London: Arena.

Stewart, D. (2009) 'Drug use and perceived treatment need among newly sentenced prisoners in England and Wales', *Addiction, 104*, 243–7.

Stokes, G., Chalk P. and Gillen, K. (eds) (2001) *Drugs and Democracy: In Search of New Directions*. Melbourne: Melbourne University Press.

Storr, A. (2008) *Churchill's Black Dog and Other Phenomena of the Human Mind*. London: Harpercollins.

Strang, J. and Gossop, M. (eds) (2005a) *Heroin Addiction and the British System (Vol. One): Origins and Evolution*. London: Routledge.

Strang, J. and Gossop, M. (eds) (2005b) *Heroin Addiction and the British System (Vol. Two)*. Abingdon: Routledge.

Sullivan, R.J. and Hagen, E.H. (2002) 'Psychotropic substance-seeking: evolutionary pathology or adaptation?', *Addiction, 97*(4), 389–400.

The Academy of Medical Sciences (2007) *Identifying the Environmental Causes of Disease: How Should We Decide What to Believe and When to Take Action?* London: The Academy of Medical Sciences.

The Academy of Medical Sciences (2008) *Brain Science, Addiction and Drugs*. London: The Academy of Medical Sciences.

The Royal Society for the Encouragement of Arts, Manufactures and Commerce (2007) *Drugs-facing Facts: The Report of the RSA Commission on Illegal Drugs, Communities and Public Policy*. London: RSA.

Thom, B. (1999) *Dealing With Drink: Alcohol and Social Policy from Treatment to Management*. London: Free Association Books.

Tirapu-Ustarroz, J., Perez-Sayes, G., Erekatxo-Bilbao, M. and Pelegrin-Valero, C. (2007) 'What is Theory of Mind?', *Review of Neurology, 44*(8), 479–89.

Todd, J., Green, G., Harrison, M., Ikuesen, B., Self, C., Baldacchino, S. and Sherwood, S. (2004) 'Defining dual diagnosis of mental illness and substance misuse: some methodological issues', *Journal of Psychiatric and Mental Health Nursing, 11*, 48–54.

United Nations Office of Drugs and Crime (2006) *World Drug Report Vol 1 Analysis*. New York.

United Nations Office of Drugs and Crime (2007) www.incb.org/incb/convention_1961.html Retrieved 18 December 2007.

United Nations Office of Drugs and Crime (2008a) 'Reducing the harm of drug use and dependence'. www.unodc.org/ddt-training/treatment/VOLUME%20D/Topic%204/1.VolD_Topic4_Harm_Reduction.pdf Retrieved 28 October 2009.

United Nations Office of Drugs and Crime (2009) The Single Convention on Narcotic Drugs 1961. www.incb.org/incb/convention_1961.html Retrieved 8 October 2009.

United Nations Office of Drugs and Crime (2009a) Convention on Psychotropic Substances 1971. www.incb.org/incb/convention_1961.html Retrieved 8 September 2009.

United Nations Office of Drugs and Crime (2009b) Conventions Against the Illicit Traffic in Narcotics and Psychotropic Substances. www.incb.org/incb/convention_1961.html Retrieved 8 October 2009.

UKATT Research Group (2001) United Kingdom Alcohol Treatment Trial (UKATT) www.bangor.ac.uk/imscar/project_info/ukatt.php.en Retrieved 15 October 2009.

United Nations Office of Drugs and Crime (2008b) 'Reducing the adverse health and social consequences of drug abuse: A comprehensive approach'. http://www.unodc.org/pdf/india/Reducing_adverse_consequences_drug_abuse.pdf Retrieved 28 October 2009.

UKATT Research Team (2001) 'United Kingdom Alcohol Treatment Trial (UKATT): hypotheses, design and methods', *Alcohol and Alcoholism, 36*(1), 11–21.

Volkow, N. and Fowler, J. (2000) 'Addiction, a disease of compulsion and drive: involvement of the orbitofrontal cortex', *Cerebral Cortex, 10*(3), 318–25.

Wanigaratne, S. (2006) 'Psychology of addiction', *Psychiatry, 5*(12), 455–60.

Weinberg, B. and Bealer, B. (2001) *The World of Caffeine: The Science and Culture of the World's Most Popular Drug*. London: Routledge.

West, R. (2001) 'Theories of addiction', *Addiction, 96*, 3–13.

West, R. (2006) *Theory of Addiction*. Oxford: Blackwell Publishing, Addiction Press.

Westerberg, V. (1998) 'What predicts success?' In W. Miller and N. Heather (eds), *Treating Addictive Behaviors*. New York: Plenum Press. pp. 301–16.

White, H.R. and Jackson, K. (2004) 'Social and psychological influences on emerging adult drinking behavior', *Alcohol Research & Health, 28*(4), 182–90.

White, W. (2004) 'Addiction recovery mutual aid groups: an enduring international phenomenon'. *Addiction 99*, 532–8.

Widerker, D. and McKenna, M. (eds) (2006) *Moral Responsibility and Alternate Possibilities*. Basingstoke: Ashgate.

Wilson, E.O. (1975) *Sociobiology: The New Synthesis*. Cambridge, MA: The Belknap Press of Harvard University Press.

Wilson, T., Holt, T. and Greenhalgh, T. (2001) 'Complexity and clinical care', *British Medical Journal, 323*(22 September), 685–8.

Yalom, I. (1980) *Existential Psychotherapy*. New York: Basic Books.

Yalom, I. (2005) *The Theory and Practice of Group Psychotherapy* (5th edition). New York: Basic Books.

Zador, D. (2005) 'Last call for injectable opiate maintenance'. In J. Strang and M. Gossop (eds), *Heroin Addiction and the British System Volume 2*. Abingdon: Routledge.

Index

NOTE: Page numbers in italic type refer to tables.

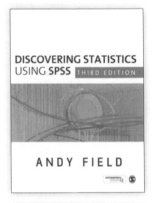
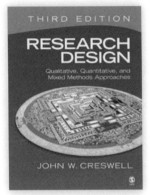
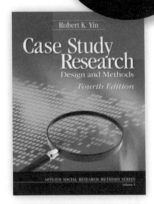
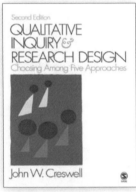
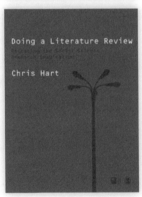
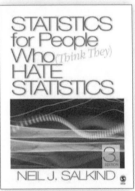
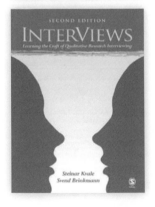
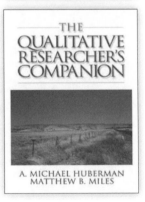
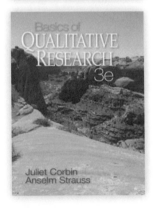
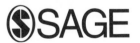

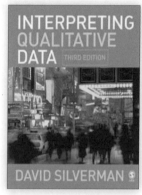
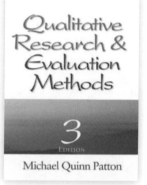
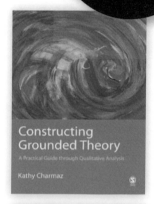
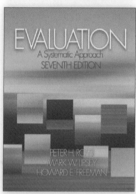
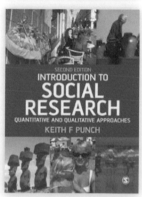
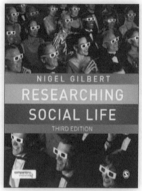
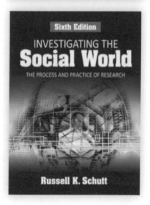
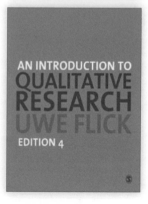
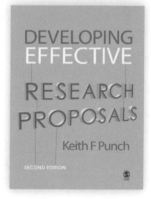
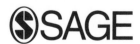